Juicing *for* beginners

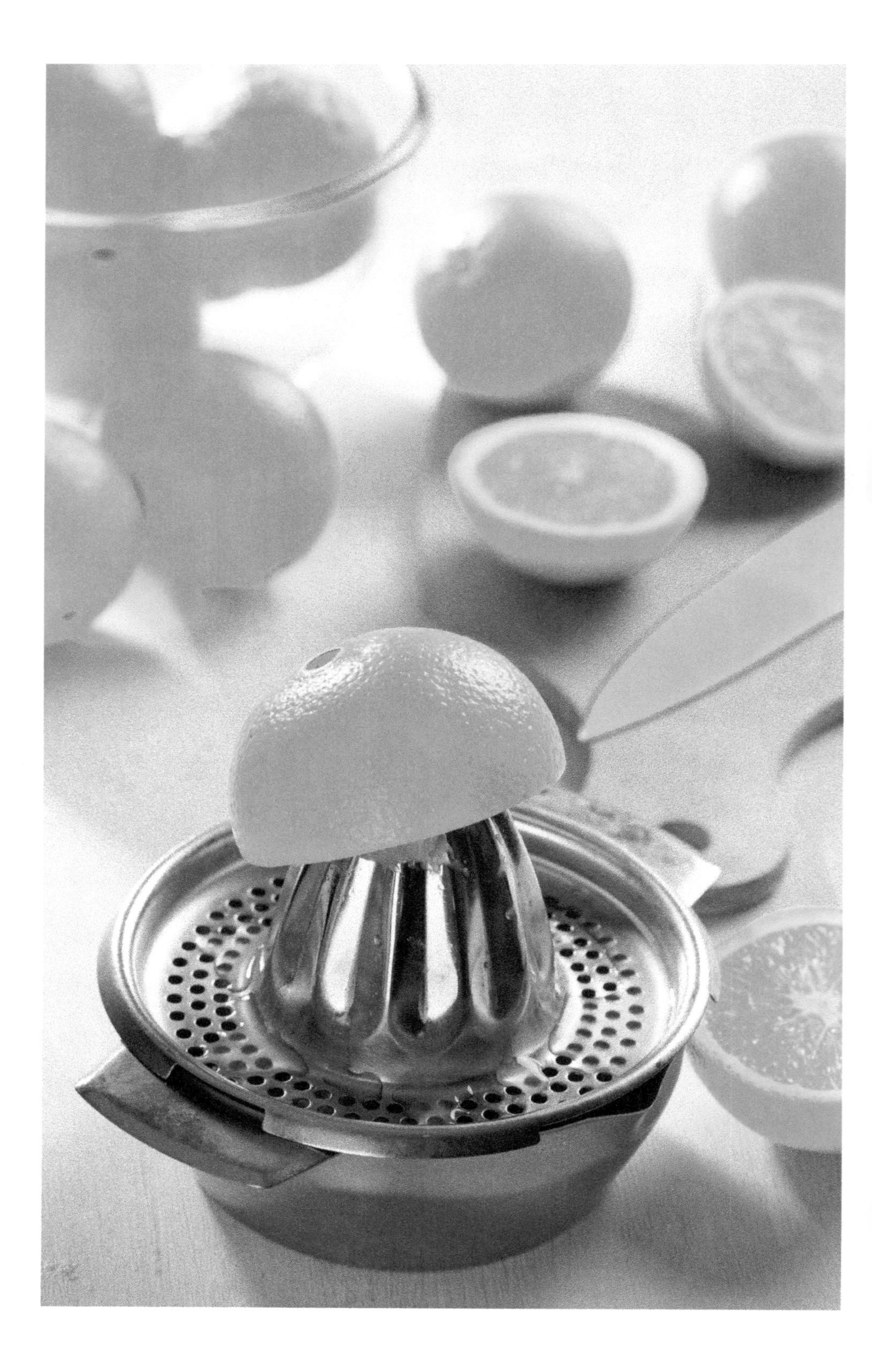

Juicing *for* beginners

THE ESSENTIAL GUIDE
to Juicing Recipes and
Juicing for Weight Loss

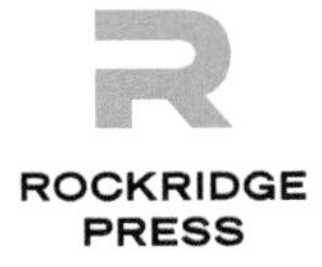

ROCKRIDGE
PRESS

For general information on our other products and services or to obtain technical support, please contact our Customer Care Department within the U.S. at (866) 744-2665, or outside the U.S. at (510) 253-0500.

Rockridge Press publishes its books in a variety of electronic and print formats. Some content that appears in print may not be available in electronic books, and vice versa.

ISBN: Print 978-1-62315-216-1 | Hard Cover 978-1-62315-415-8 | eBook 978-1-62315-217-8

Contents

Introduction

"Every person has the ability to reclaim all or some measure of their health. And every person who does that becomes a leader who inspires others."

JOE CROSS, CO-DIRECTOR AND CO-WRITER OF *FAT, SICK & NEARLY DEAD*

Joe Cross is just one of countless individuals who have transformed their health and their lives through juicing. If you are unfamiliar with the concept, you may be tempted to think that juicing is just another health and fitness trend, or some kind of fad diet. In reality, however, it is a method through which you can easily increase your daily intake of essential nutrients while also cleansing your body and boosting your weight-loss efforts. If you have ever struggled to lose weight, juicing may be the solution you've been looking for.

You don't need to follow a diet plan prescribed by some health-and-fitness guru to successfully incorporate juicing into your diet. Juicing is easy and there is no wrong way to go about it. Create your own flavor combinations using your favorite fruits and vegetables, and throw in some healthy additives to boost the nutritional value of your juices. Once you start juicing, you may find yourself wondering why you waited so long to begin.

In this book, you will find a comprehensive overview of the benefits of juicing along with 100 juicing recipes to help you begin this delicious and healthy life choice. Not only will you learn the details of how juicing can improve your health and boost your weight loss, but you will learn exactly what nutritional benefits raw fruits and vegetables have to offer. In addition to improving your overall health and wellness, juicing can also improve or even reverse symptoms of chronic diseases including diabetes, asthma, high blood pressure, and Crohn's disease. Equipped with all of this valuable information and the recipes you need to get started, you will be ready to juice right away.

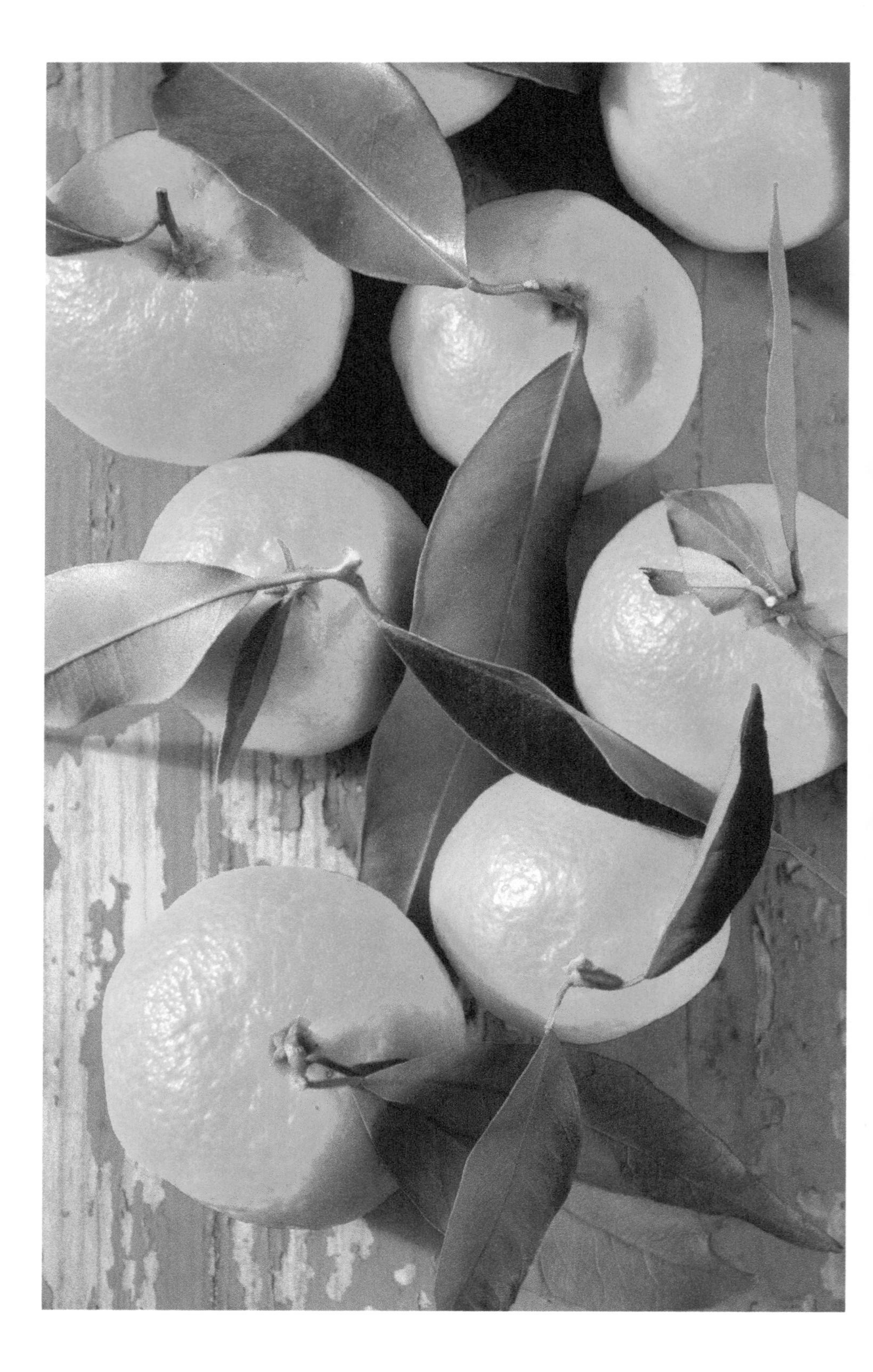

CHAPTER ONE

The Basics

"If you don't enjoy eating fresh fruits and vegetables, juicing may be a fun way to add them to your diet or to try fruits and vegetables you normally wouldn't eat."

JENNIFER K. NELSON, R.D., L.D.

What Is Juicing?

Simply put, juicing is the process of extracting juice from fruits and vegetables. Juicing can be done by hand with a citrus press or it can be done using an electric household appliance called a juicer. As a health trend, the word "juicing" typically refers to the practice of increasing your daily intake of fresh fruits and vegetables by drinking freshly pressed juices. People engage in juicing for a variety of reasons, mostly health-related. In addition to increasing your intake of healthy nutrients, juicing also provides benefits for weight loss, detoxification, and more.

Benefits of Juicing Versus Eating Raw Fruits and Vegetables

Registered dieticians and other healthcare professionals are divided on the issue of whether or not juicing is more beneficial than eating raw fruits and vegetables. While juicing certainly isn't unhealthy, there is some debate as to whether it is healthier than just eating the fruits and vegetables themselves. Jennifer K.

Nelson, a registered dietician, writes that "juicing extracts the juice from fresh fruits or vegetables . . . the resulting liquid contains most of the vitamins, minerals, and plant chemicals (phytonutrients) found in the whole fruit." As many detractors of the juicing trend are keen to point out, however, a significant portion of the fiber content of fruits and vegetables is lost during the juicing process.

In order to understand the differences between juicing and eating raw fruits and vegetables, you need to know the basics about how a juicer works. A juicer is a kitchen appliance that takes the work out of extracting the juice from fresh fruits and vegetables. These devices are motor-operated, and they come in a variety of sizes. Though the mechanics of different models may vary, most juicers require you to push the raw fruits and vegetables through a feed tube. Inside, the appliance extracts the juice from the plant fibers, separating out the seeds, skin, and pulp. The fresh juice then exits the machine through a spout and into the desired glass or container.

For many people, making use of a juicer is a quick and easy way to boost the daily intake of fruits and vegetables. While it is true that some of the fiber content of the raw fruits and vegetables is lost during juicing, there are many unique benefits that juicing provides over eating raw fruits and vegetables. These include:

- Juicing is an excellent alternative if you do not normally like eating raw fruits and vegetables.
- The results are delicious—you can even disguise the flavor of vegetables by combining them with your favorite fruits.
- Juicing is a quick and easy process; the resulting juice can be taken with you for an on-the-go meal.
- Adding some of the pulp to your pressed juice will help restore some of its fiber content.
- Juicing does not require you to peel or chop the produce before using it (depending on the type of juicer you buy).
- Homemade juices have a fresh-squeezed taste; store-bought juices simply can't compare.
- Juicing is a great way to help your kids get the vitamins and minerals they need from fruits and vegetables.
- Leftover pulp from juicing can be used in baked goods, such as muffins, or as a base for homemade stocks and broths.

- Juicing is an economical way to make use of fruits and vegetables that are about to spoil.

Making Your Own Juice

While the process of juicing is as easy as feeding fresh fruits and vegetables through your juicer, there are a few things you may need to do before you take that first step. You do not need to worry about peeling or chopping your produce, but you should take the time to wash it first. Even if you purchase organic produce, it could still carry bacteria. Once you've thoroughly washed the produce, you need to prepare your juicer. These preparations will vary depending on the type of juicer. If your juicer has a pulp basket or canister, lining it with a plastic bag will make cleanup easier.

Next, turn the juicer on and feed the produce through it on the speed recommended in the manufacturer's instructions. Remember, you don't always need to peel or chop the produce, but you may need to cut it in half or tear large leaves into smaller pieces for them to fit into the feed tube. Refer to the directions provided with your juicer to determine the right speed for different types of produce. (Softer foods like berries may require a low speed while hard produce such as beets or apples will require a higher speed.) After you finish feeding the produce through the juicer, check the pulp basket or canister. If you find chunks of unprocessed produce, or if the pulp is still wet, feed it through the machine again to extract as much juice as possible.

Once you've finished, you can enjoy your delicious beverage. It is important to drink your juice as soon as possible after pressing it because, like all fresh foods exposed to air, it could develop bacteria if you let it sit for too long. If you make more juice than you can consume at one time, store the extra in an airtight container in the refrigerator for up to forty-eight hours. Glass containers are best because plastic may contain BPA (bisphenol A), a chemical that can cause serious health problems. If you do store your juice, fill the container as full as you can manage—over time, excess oxygen in the container may deplete the nutrients in your juice.

Juicing for Detoxification

If you are familiar with the juicing trend, you may have also heard of a juice cleanse. Also known as a juice fast, it involves consuming nothing but fruit and vegetable juices for a predetermined length of time. Though long-term fasting of this kind is generally not recommended, a three- to five-day juice cleanse may provide numerous health benefits. Skeptics of juice cleansing suggest that there is no scientific evidence to support the idea that consuming fresh fruit and vegetable juices will rid your body of toxins. While juicing may not be a magical solution to the world's health problems, it does provide a number of benefits that may help to cleanse and detoxify your body.

The modern Western diet is centered on processed foods, which are loaded with artificial preservatives, flavors, and other toxins. Thankfully, the human body is designed to filter out and eliminate these toxins; however, the average Western diet creates a toxic load much higher than the body is capable of handling. Your liver, kidneys, lungs, and skin are the primary detoxifying organs in your body, and when they become overloaded, your body may begin storing excess toxins in your fat cells and tissues. Over time, your body will become toxic and you may experience a number of negative side effects, including indigestion, allergies, constipation, dry hair and skin, breakouts, and more.

It is important to understand that fresh fruit and vegetable juices will not magically make the toxins in your body disappear. Juicing can, however, play a role in naturally detoxifying your body. Engaging in a juice cleanse means that you will stop poisoning your body with toxic-laden processed foods, replacing them instead with nutrient-rich juices. If, after you complete your juice cleanse, you continue to avoid processed foods and maintain a habit of consuming fresh fruits and vegetables, your body will naturally begin to recover from its toxic overload. By reducing your intake of toxins, your body will be able to focus on stored toxins and flush them from your system, which will result in improved overall health.

Choosing a Juicer

Choosing a juicer can be a confusing process if you don't already understand the basics. Before you go shopping for your new juicer, take the time to learn about the three different types so you can decide which option is best for you. The three main types of juicers are: centrifugal juicers, masticating juicers, and triturating juicers. Each type has its own list of pros and cons, so in order to select the right one for your situation, you need to think about what features you want. You should also decide what price range you are willing to consider, because juicers can be quite expensive.

Centrifugal Juicers

A centrifugal juicer is perhaps the simplest type of juicer. For one thing, it is easy to operate and easy to clean. Also, these juicers utilize a grated basket that acts as a spinning blade, grinding the produce and extracting the juice. The pulp remains in the basket while the juice passes through the holes and exits the appliance through the spout. These juicers work very quickly and are one of the most affordable options, but they are not well equipped to handle very hard produce or pitted fruits.

Masticating Juicers

A masticating juicer operates more slowly than a centrifugal juicer. These juicers work by kneading and grinding the material in the feed chute, squeezing the juice out into a container. The benefit of this type of juicer is that it operates at a lower speed than other juicers, which means that it produces less heat. Because the juicer doesn't get very hot, fewer enzymes are killed, so the juice should not oxidize very much, giving it a longer shelf life.

Triturating Juicers

A triturating juicer is a twin-gear juicer that utilizes a two-step juicing process. When produce is fed through the juicer, it is first crushed and then it is pressed. These appliances may be a little pricier, but they are the most efficient. They also produce little heat, which is ideal for preserving enzymes and limiting oxidization.

Questions to Ask When Choosing a Juicer

Once you've decided on the type of juicer you want, you then have to sort through the various brands and models. Asking yourself these questions may help you narrow down your options:

What kinds of produce do you plan to juice?

Certain juicers are more capable than others of handling hard fruits such as apples or leafy vegetables.

How much noise does the juicer make?

If you plan to make your juice before others in your household are awake, you might want to choose a model that runs quietly.

How much heat does the juicer produce?

Store-bought juices are pasteurized, which destroys the natural enzymes contained in the juice. To prevent this from occurring in your own juice, you may want to select a juicer that doesn't produce much heat.

It is easy to clean?

If you plan to use your juicer on a daily basis, you don't want to spend all of your time cleaning it. Choose a model that is easy to disassemble, wash, and put back together.

Does it take up a lot of space?

If you have plenty of extra cabinet space or a storage closet, this may not matter much. However, if you plan to leave your juicer out on the counter, you should be sure you have enough room.

What is the capacity of the juicer?

Juicers come in all different sizes—if you are juicing only for yourself, you may not have to worry about capacity. If you are juicing for the family or plan to make extra juice to store, you may need a larger juicer.

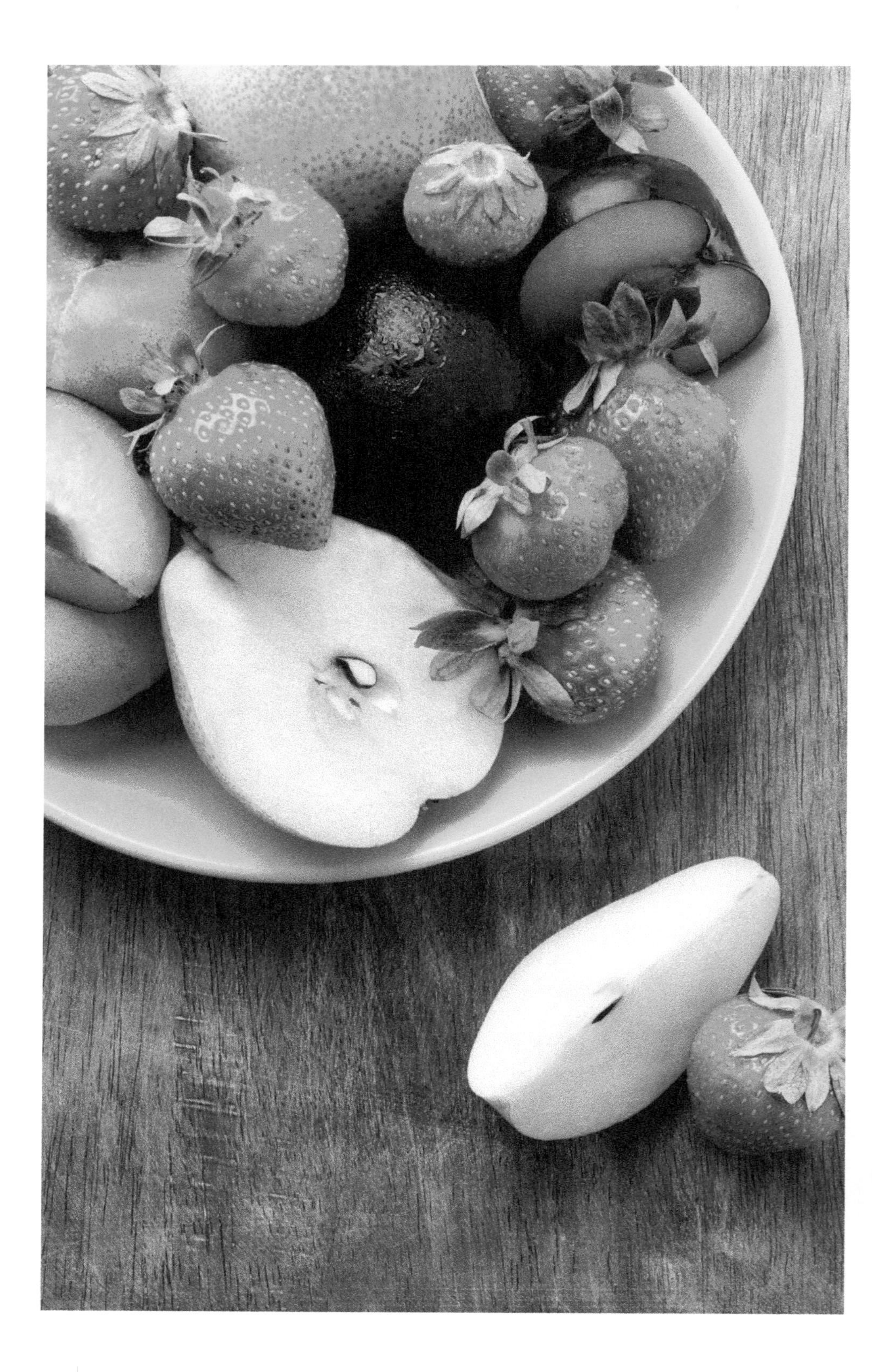

CHAPTER TWO

Fruits

> "Eating a diet with plenty of fruits and vegetables has been linked to improved health, and for good reason . . . Fruits are loaded with vitamins, minerals, fiber, and antioxidants, which have been shown to protect against chronic diseases such as heart disease and cancer. They are also low in calories, making them a great choice for your waistline."
>
> LISA R. YOUNG, PH.D, R.D., AUTHOR OF *THE PORTION TELLER PLAN*

You will find the following fruits as ingredients in the healthy juice recipes in this book:

- Apple
- Banana
- Black cherry
- Blueberry
- Grape
- Kiwi
- Lime
- Melon
- Papaya
- Peach
- Avocado
- Blackberry
- Blood orange
- Cantaloupe
- Grapefruit
- Lemon
- Mango
- Orange
- Passion fruit
- Pear

- Pineapple
- Pomegranate
- Raspberry
- Strawberry
- Tangerine

Health Benefits of Fruits

Apple: Apples contain an antioxidant called quercetin, which helps to reduce LDL (bad) cholesterol levels. These fruits are also rich in a soluble fiber called pectin, which may help flush toxic heavy metals from the body.

Avocado: Avocados are an excellent source of heart-healthy fats (monounsaturated fats). In addition, avocados provide potassium to regulate blood pressure, vitamin K to promote bone health, and plant-based protein.

Banana: Bananas are rich in B vitamins, which help promote healthy sleep patterns and reduce mood swings and irritability. This fruit also provides plenty of vitamin C in addition to potassium and magnesium, all of which help to replenish the body's store of electrolytes. Bananas are also naturally sweet—they can be pureed and blended into any of your favorite juices.

Blackberry: In addition to being an excellent source of vitamin C, blackberries contain high levels of calcium, potassium, iron, and fiber. Berries like blackberries contain the highest levels of antioxidants of any fruit.

Black Cherry: Cherries are an excellent source of iron, which helps the body produce healthy blood cells. These fruits also contain an anti-cancer compound called ellagic acid, and have high levels of vitamins A and C. In addition to these nutrients, cherries also possess antioxidant, anti-inflammatory, and antibacterial properties.

Blood Orange: Blood oranges are a variety of orange known for their crimson-colored flesh. This unique color is due to high levels of anthocyanins, a type of antioxidant pigment—their presence makes blood oranges richer in antioxidants than other oranges. Blood oranges are also a good source of dietary fiber, vitamin C, calcium, and folate.

Blueberry: Like apples, blueberries contain pectin as well as flavonoids, which may help reduce your risk for type 2 diabetes. Blueberries are also rich in vitamin C, potassium, and tannins, which have antiviral and antibacterial properties. Additionally, blueberries contain manganese, which contributes to healthy bone growth.

Cantaloupe: Cantaloupes are round melons with a bright orange flesh that is bursting with nutrients. Though full of juice and sweet flavor, cantaloupe is low in calories, and an excellent source of folic acid, beta-carotene, fiber, potassium, and vitamin C. Unlike many fruits and vegetables, cantaloupe also contains complex B vitamins.

Grape: Grapes are rich in a number of vitamins, including A, B, and C, in addition to minerals such as calcium, iron, phosphorus, magnesium, potassium, and selenium. Grapes also contain flavonoids, a powerful antioxidant that can help repair damage caused by free radicals—this property makes grapes an excellent anti-aging aid.

Grapefruit: Like all citrus fruits, grapefruit is an excellent source of vitamin C. Grapefruit also contains limonene, a compound that may help reduce the risk of breast cancer. Additionally, grapefruits are a great source of soluble fiber, which may help lower unhealthy blood cholesterol levels.

Kiwi: Kiwi is an excellent source of vitamin C, which helps to heal wounds and keep your teeth and gums healthy. These fruits also contain vitamin K, vitamin E, folate, copper, and potassium. The enzymes found in kiwi have been shown to soothe digestive issues and may reduce the appearance of wrinkles.

Lemon: Lemon is often referred to as the most powerful fruit for detoxification. It has been linked to cancer prevention, relief from digestive issues, and reduced risk for heart disease and stroke. Lemons are rich in calcium, magnesium, potassium, and phosphorus.

Lime: Limes are very similar to lemons in their nutritional properties. These fruits are a good source of vitamin C, vitamin B6, folate, and potassium. Limes also contain flavonoids, a powerful antioxidant, and various other phytonutrients.

Mango: Mangoes contain both vitamin A and vitamin C, which make them very beneficial for strengthening the immune system. Mangoes are a good source of potassium, which has been shown to regulate heart rate and blood pressure. They have also been linked to reduced risk for certain types of cancer.

Melon: Melons, such as honeydew and watermelon, possess both antioxidant and anti-cancer properties. These fruits contain adenosine, a naturally occurring chemical that may reduce the risk for cancer and stroke.

Orange: Oranges are known for their vitamin C content, but they actually contain more than 170 different phytonutrients. These fruits have been shown to help shrink tumors, prevent blood clots, and reduce inflammation.

Papaya: Papayas are known for their antioxidant and anti-cancer properties. These fruits contain powerful enzymes that help to reduce constipation and promote healthy digestion. Additionally, papayas are a good source of potassium and vitamins A and C.

Passion Fruit: Passion fruit is a very aromatic fruit with a unique flavor. They are an excellent source of dietary fiber, vitamin A, vitamin C, and beta-carotene. Passion fruit is also rich in potassium, which may help regulate blood pressure and reduce the risk for cardiovascular disease.

Peach: In addition to their sweet flavor, peaches are also known for being an excellent source of both vitamin A and potassium. These fruits also contain boron and niacin, or vitamin B3, which has been shown to reduce the risk for cardiovascular disease.

Pear: Pears are an excellent source of dietary fiber, vitamin C, boron, and potassium. These fruits have been used for a variety of benefits, including as a diuretic, a cleanser, and a digestive aid.

Pineapple: Pineapples are a good source of iron, potassium, and vitamin C. These fruits also contain bromelain and other anti-inflammatory compounds, which help to promote joint health. Pineapple has also been used as a natural diuretic and a mild laxative.

Pomegranate: Pomegranates are an excellent fruit for cleansing and detoxing the body. These fruits contain vitamin C, magnesium, potassium, and beta-carotene—they have also been identified as the third-highest fruit source of antioxidants. Pomegranates contain lycopene and other phytonutrients that may help reduce the risk for prostate cancer.

Raspberry: In addition to being rich in vitamins C, K, and E, raspberries also contain folate, manganese, copper, and iron. Raspberries have been shown to help lower LDL (bad) cholesterol and to inhibit the growth of certain cancers.

Strawberry: Like most berries, strawberries are a good source of vitamin C, which helps to heal wounds and improve gum and teeth health. Strawberries are also known to have antiviral, antioxidant, and anti-cancer properties. These berries have also been linked to lowering LDL (bad) cholesterol, suppressing colon cancer, and protecting against Alzheimer's disease.

Tangerine: Tangerines are a good source of calcium, copper, magnesium, potassium, and beta-carotene. These fruits also contain sulfur, which helps promote detoxification of the liver. Additionally, tangerines have been shown to have antibacterial, anti-cancer, diuretic, and decongestant properties.

See the Nutritional Information for Fruits chart at the back of the book for the breakdown of the calories, protein, carbs, fats, and fiber for the fruits (serving size = 100 grams) mentioned in this chapter.

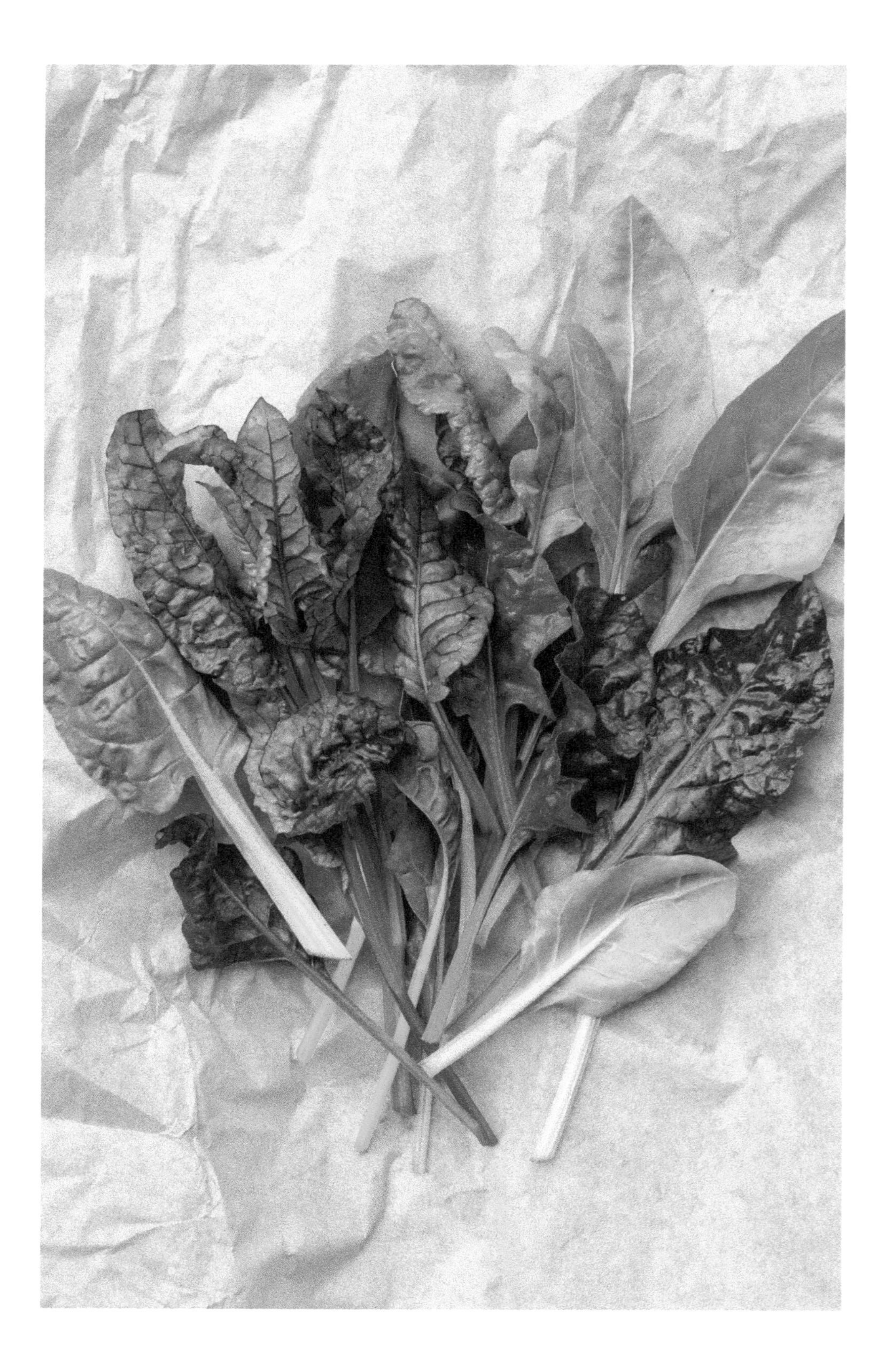

CHAPTER THREE

Vegetables

"Greens have more valuable nutrients than any other food group on the planet . . . Blending helps make greens' full spectrum of nutrition readily available to the body . . . helping your body absorb the maximum amount of nutrition from your greens."

KIMBERLY SNYDER, C.N., AUTHOR OF *THE BEAUTY DETOX SOLUTION*

You will find the following vegetables as ingredients in the healthy juice recipes in this book:

- Arugula
- Asparagus
- Beet
- Bell Pepper
- Bok Choy
- Broccoli
- Brussels Sprout
- Cabbage
- Carrot
- Cauliflower
- Celery
- Cilantro
- Collard Greens
- Cucumber
- Dandelion Greens
- Fennel
- Garlic
- Ginger
- Kale
- Mint
- Parsley
- Parsnip

- Pumpkin
- Spinach
- Sweet Potato
- Tomato
- Romaine Lettuce
- Summer Squash
- Swiss Chard
- Zucchini

Health Benefits of Vegetables

Arugula: Arugula is a leafy green and a cruciferous vegetable, which means that it is rich in antioxidants and flavonoids that may help reduce your risk for cancer. Arugula is also a good source for vitamins A, C, and K and a variety of essential minerals.

Asparagus: Asparagus is an excellent source of folate, which is vital for fetal development. This vegetable is also packed with antioxidants, which have been shown to reduce the appearance of aging and to slow cognitive decline. Asparagus also contains dietary fiber, chromium, and vitamins A, C, E, and K.

Beet: Beets and beet greens are an excellent source of iron, choline, iodine, manganese, potassium, and vitamins A and C. Additionally, studies have shown that beets help to oxygenate the blood, enhancing performance while exercising.

Bell Pepper: Red, green, and yellow bell peppers contain high levels of vitamin C, which is essential for healing wounds and for maintaining eye and gum health. They also contain vitamin A, which is a key contributor to skin and eye health.

Bok Choy: A type of leafy Chinese cabbage, bok choy is rich in a variety of phytonutrients, vitamins, and minerals. This vegetable is a good source of antioxidants, which combined with fiber and various vitamins, makes bok choy an anti-cancer and cholesterol-reducing food.

Broccoli: Like arugula, broccoli is a cruciferous vegetable and an excellent source of dietary fiber. It contains vitamin C, which helps promote healing, as well as vitamin E, which may help reduce your risk for certain cancers. Broccoli is also rich in iron, potassium, calcium, selenium, zinc, and sulfur.

Brussels Sprout: These vegetables are rich in dietary fiber, folate, potassium, and manganese. A single cup of Brussels sprouts also contains more than 100 percent of your daily recommended intake of both vitamins C and K. Brussels sprouts have been linked to cancer prevention and have also been shown to support detoxification.

Cabbage: Cabbage is one of few vegetables that naturally contain vitamin E. This vegetable is also rich in sulfur, which has been shown to help purify the blood and detoxify the liver. Cabbage also contains antibacterial, antioxidant, and anti-inflammatory properties.

Carrot: Carrots are one of the most readily available vegetables, and they are also incredibly rich in vitamins and minerals. Carrots are a great source of vitamins A, B, and C as well as iron, calcium, potassium, and sodium. Carrots also contain beta-carotene and carotenoids, which help reduce the risk for cancer, cardiovascular disease, and macular degeneration.

Cauliflower: Cauliflower is an extremely versatile vegetable that is also rich in a number of nutrients. High in B vitamins, phosphorus, potassium, manganese, and vitamin K, this vegetable is very nutrient dense. Cauliflower is also a good source of antioxidants as well as glucosinolates, which help support the liver's detox abilities.

Celery: A very low-calorie food, celery is rich in a variety of vitamins and minerals. The silicon content of celery helps to strengthen joints and bones, while iron and magnesium help support blood health. Celery has also been shown to have diuretic and anti-cancer properties.

Cilantro: Cilantro is an herb that is incredibly rich in antioxidants that can help lower your LDL (bad) cholesterol and raise your good (HDL) cholesterol levels. This herb contains numerous vitamins, including folic acid, niacin, beta-carotene, and vitamins A, C, and K. There is also research to suggest that cilantro may be beneficial in managing Alzheimer's disease.

Collard Greens: Collard greens are an excellent source of vitamin C, manganese, chlorophyll, and beta-carotene. They have both antioxidant and anti-cancer properties. They may also be the strongest of all vegetables in lowering unhealthy cholesterol levels.

Cucumber: Cucumbers are an excellent source of potassium and phytosterols, both of which help to lower cholesterol. These vegetables have a high water content, which makes them great for juicing. They are also a good source of B vitamins and may help control blood pressure.

Dandelion Greens: Though it may sound odd to eat them, dandelion greens are actually incredibly healthy. These greens are an excellent source of vitamin K, which helps to support blood and bone health. Dandelion greens also contain nutrients that contribute to liver and gallbladder health.

Fennel: Fennel is particularly beneficial for the digestive system. This herb contains calcium, folate, potassium, magnesium, phosphorus, iron, and copper. It is also a good source of vitamins C and B5.

Garlic: Garlic is known for its antimicrobial, antibiotic, and anti-cancer properties. This allium helps to lower blood cholesterol levels and to regulate blood sugar. Garlic also contains a variety of vitamins, minerals, and antioxidants, which make it valuable for boosting the immune system.

Ginger: Ginger is an excellent food for detoxing—it cleanses the body and helps to support healthy digestion. Ginger also has antinausea, anti-inflammatory, and antioxidant properties.

Green Onion: Green onions are also called scallions or spring onions, and they contain a variety of vitamins and minerals as well as other phytochemicals. These vegetables contain vitamins K and C, which help to support bone health, as well as vitamin A for eye health. Green onions are also a good source of various phytochemicals like quercetin and anthocyanins, which boost immune system health.

Kale: Kale is the highest vegetable source of vitamin K, which may help reduce the risk for certain cancers. This leafy vegetable is also a good source of calcium, iron, chlorophyll, and vitamins C and A. Kale is very nutrient dense, providing many healthy minerals, including iron, potassium, phosphorus, and manganese.

Mint: Mint is an herb that helps to soothe both indigestion and inflammation—its scent alone can stimulate the salivary glands, encouraging the production of enzymes that aid digestion. Mint is also a good source of plant-based omega-3 fatty acids, which support healthy hair, skin, and nails.

Parsley: This herb is one of the highest natural sources for vitamin C. Parsley is rich in folate, which helps to prevent certain cancers and may also improve heart health. It also has diuretic properties, which means that it helps the body flush excess water.

Parsnip: Parsnips are known for their anti-cancer and anti- inflammatory properties. These vegetables contain high levels of vitamins C and E as well as protein, iron, and calcium. Parsnips have also been used as a natural diuretic and detoxifier.

Pumpkin: Pumpkin has been shown to reduce inflammation and may also reduce your risk for prostate cancer. This vegetable is high in vitamins C and E as well as copper, iron, and potassium. The phytochemicals present in pumpkin have also been shown to have a favorable effect on insulin and glucose levels in diabetes lab models.

Radish: Radishes are the roots of cruciferous vegetables, and they are an excellent source of vitamins and minerals. The leaves of the plant contain more protein, calcium, and vitamin C than the roots, and they have often been used to fight cancer, treat kidney problems, and soothe skin irritation. Radishes are also rich in vitamin C, folic acid, and anthocyanins, which make them effective as a cancer-fighting food.

Romaine Lettuce: While some lettuces (like iceberg) are fairly low in nutrients, that is not the case with romaine lettuce. This lettuce is incredibly rich in vitamins A, K, and C as well as potassium, iron, magnesium, and manganese.

Spinach: Spinach is a great source of vitamins A, C, and E, and it also contains high levels of calcium, iron, potassium, and protein. Additionally, spinach contains choline, a B-complex vitamin that supports healthy cognitive function. The iron content in spinach helps to build healthy blood cells.

Summer Squash: Summer squash is very low in calories but rich in vitamins. These vegetables contain vitamins C and A as well as magnesium, copper, riboflavin, and phosphorus. Summer squash is also a good source of antioxidants, which help to repair damage from free radicals.

Sweet Potato: Sweet potatoes have been identified as beneficial for eye health, detoxification, and digestive support. High in copper, iron, magnesium, manganese, and other nutrients, sweet potatoes also have anti-cancer properties.

Swiss Chard: A leafy green vegetable, Swiss chard (and other chards), is considered one of the healthiest vegetables available. Chards are rich in dietary fiber and protein in addition to containing high levels of vitamins A, K, and C.

Tomato: Tomatoes are a good source of vitamin C, potassium, copper, iron, and magnesium. They are known to contain over nine thousand phytonutrients, including the antioxidant lycopene, which has been linked to cancer prevention and improved mental and physical health.

Zucchini: Zucchini is a good source of copper, iron, magnesium, manganese, phosphorus, potassium, and vitamin C.This vegetable is also a good source of vitamin A and niacin (vitamin B3), which has been linked to reduced risk for cardiovascular disease.

See the Nutritional Information for Vegetables chart at the back of the book for the breakdown of the calories, protein, carbs, fats, and fiber for the vegetables (serving size = 100 grams) mentioned in this chapter.

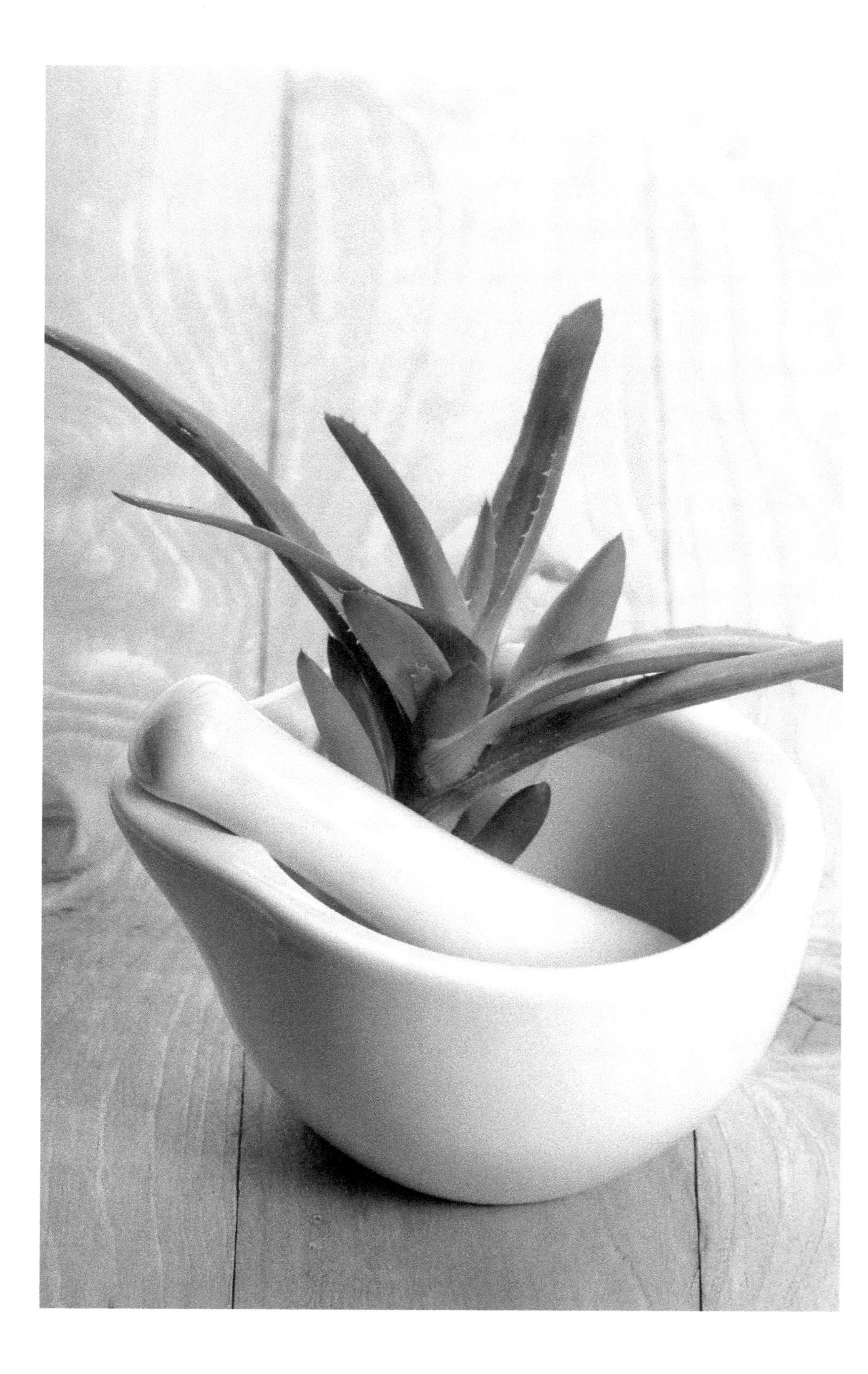

CHAPTER FOUR

Additives for Variety

"When you consistently drink fresh raw juice, especially vegetable juice that includes plenty of dark leafy greens, along with eating lots of vegetables and fruit and a very healthy diet, your whole internal environment changes. Juice, which is rich in antioxidants, cleanses the body of stored wastes and toxins that interfere with the proper functioning of cells and organs. . . . A healthy, vibrant internal environment is a key to optimum health."

CHERIE CALBOM, M.S., AUTHOR OF
THE JUICE LADY'S GUIDE TO JUICING FOR HEALTH

You will find the following additives as ingredients in the healthy juice recipes in this book:

- Aloe vera
- Chlorella
- Essential oils
- Flaxseed
- Hempseed
- Herbal extracts
- Probiotic capsules
- Spirulina
- Vitamin B12
- Wheatgrass
- Whey powder

The Health Benefits of Additives

Aloe Vera: The juice derived from the aloe vera plant can help to reduce inflammation and internal stress. It also has antifungal, antiviral, and antibacterial properties. Because it contains a variety of vitamins and minerals, aloe vera can also help boost your immune system.

Chlorella: A type of alga, chlorella is rich in a variety of nutrients, including protein, chlorophyll, iron, zinc, and vitamin B12. This additive can help to lower unhealthy cholesterol levels and may also boost the immune system. Additionally, chlorella may help detoxify the body and regulate your digestion.

Essential Oils: Essential fatty acids (EFAs) can be derived from a variety of plant-based oils from seeds, nuts, and avocados. These fatty acids are essential for healthy hair and skin. They may also help regulate your metabolism and support healthy weight loss.

Flaxseed: Flaxseed can be incorporated into juicing in either whole seed or ground form—you can also use flaxseed oil. These seeds are rich in omega-3 fatty acids, fiber, and protein. Flaxseed also contains lignans, a type of chemical compound that acts as an antioxidant in the body.

Hempseed: Hempseed is the seed of the cannabis plant and is rich in fiber and healthy oils. Hempseed contains essential fatty acids, linoleic acid, and protein. These seeds are a more complete protein than milk, meat, and eggs. Hempseed also contains fiber, vitamin A, iron, and sodium.

Herbal Extracts: Liquid herbal extracts are an excellent addition to juices because even a small amount can provide a variety of vitamins and minerals. Unlike capsules and tablets, herbal extracts are in the ideal form to be absorbed and digested by the body. Though herbal extracts often have a bitter or powerful flavor, this can be disguised by mixing them into healthy juices.

Probiotic Capsules: Probiotics are living microorganisms that help to restore and improve healthy digestive function. In combination with fruits and vegetables, probiotics can help flush toxins out of your system. To use probiotic capsules for juicing, prepare the juice, and then break open a capsule and stir in the contents.

Spirulina: Typically used in powder form, spirulina is made from algae, which are rich in both protein and essential amino acids, making spirulina a healthy additive for juices. Spirulina also contains calcium and a variety of other minerals that boost thyroid function.

Vitamin B12: This vitamin isn't something that is found in plant foods—it is actually produced by microorganisms that can be found in soil or on certain plants, like wheatgrass. Vitamin B12 deficiency can cause a number of significant health problems, including memory and hearing loss, and vision impairment.

Wheatgrass: Wheatgrass is derived from the wheat plant, and it can be used in either juice or powdered form. Wheatgrass is thought to have anti-cancer properties, and it may be part of an effective therapy for ulcerative colitis, indigestion, and general detoxification. It also contains vitamin B12.

Whey Powder: Whey powder is a nutritional supplement made from the proteins isolated from milk. This supplement can be added to juicing recipes to increase the protein content. It may also be fortified with other vitamins and minerals, depending on the brand.

See the Nutritional Information for Additives chart at the back of the book for the breakdown of the calories, protein, carbs, fats, and fiber for the vegetables (serving size = 28 grams) mentioned in this chapter.

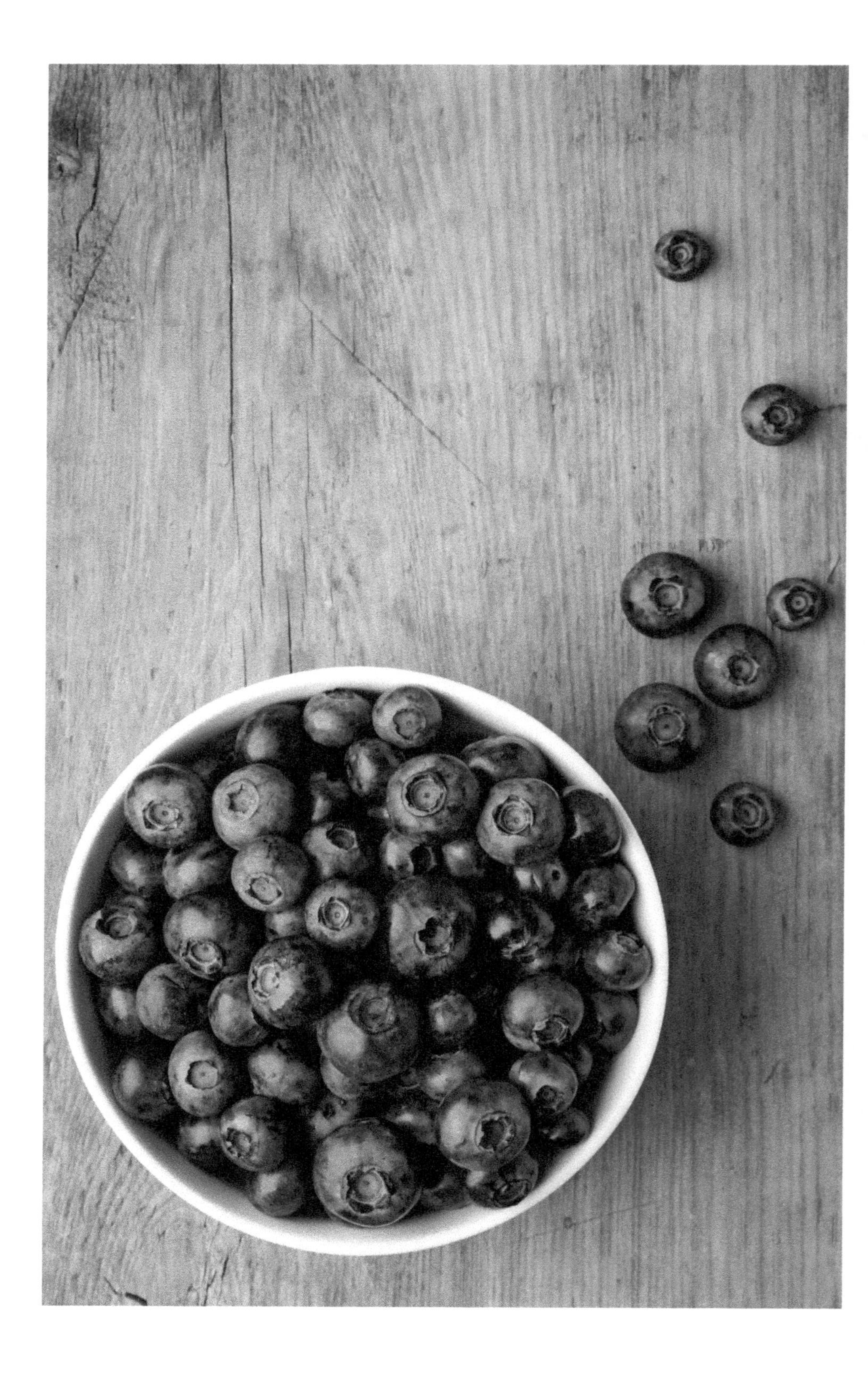

CHAPTER FIVE

Health Problems and Common Ailments

"There is fundamentally only one disease and therefore one solution. The body gets sick due to two basic things—toxicity and deficiency. If we remove the toxicity and replace any deficiencies, the vast majority of common ailments improve or go away completely . . . it really is that simple."

JASON VALE, AUTHOR OF *7 LBS IN 7 DAYS: THE JUICE MASTER DIET*

Though proponents of juicing do not claim that it is a comprehensive cure for physical ailments and serious medical conditions, that is not to say it isn't therapeutic. An article published by the American Society for Clinical Nutrition in 2005 draws a connection between the evolution of the Western diet and the proliferation of chronic disease. The authors of the article state that "the discordance between our ancient, genetically determined biology and the nutritional, cultural, and activity patterns of contemporary Western populations" has resulted in the emergence of "so-called diseases of civilization" (Cordain et al., 2005).

The Consequences of the Western Diet

Throughout the article, Cordain et al. explore the evolutionary history of the human genome and the effects of evolutionary discordance. The authors write that, through the process of natural selection, genetic traits are passed on or phased out according to their concordance with the environment. During the Paleolithic Era—a period in history that began approximately

2.6 million years ago and ended around 10,000 BCE—the environment in which humans lived remained fairly constant. With the birth of agriculture, however, that environment began to change rapidly, and the human diet underwent a drastic transformation. With improved technology, mankind was able to produce and consume foods like grains and dairy products, which had heretofore been unknown to them.

According to Cordain et al., the human genome has not evolved significantly in the centuries following the Paleolithic Era. Permanent environmental changes, however, have occurred—particularly in Western cultures where processed foods and a largely sedentary lifestyle have become the norm. Cordain et al. rite that "this evolutionary discordance manifests itself phenotypically as disease; increased morbidity and mortality; and reduced reproductive success" (2005). Chronic diseases and health problems have long been considered one of the most serious threats to public health in Western cultures; both researchers and medical professionals alike attribute a significant portion of that threat to diet.

Pre-agricultural Nutrition

Prior to the development of agriculture, humans engaged in hunter-gatherer lifestyles. Though the diets of individuals may have varied by geographical location and ecology, early human diets shared one important characteristic: they were composed of minimally processed foods derived from plants and animals. As advances in agriculture brought new food sources to the table, foods that required processing—like grains, legumes, and dairy products—started to replace fresh fruits and vegetables as staples of the typical human diet. As cited by Cordain et al., processed foods including "dairy products, cereals, refined sugars, refined vegetables oils, and alcohol make up 72.1 percent of the total daily energy consumed by people in the United States" (2005). It is not difficult to make the connection between the drastic decline in the nutritional value of the Western diet and the significant increase in health problems and chronic disease.

Health Problems Common in Western Culture

Modern Western cultures are stricken with dozens of chronic diseases that affect a significant portion of the population. An estimated 65 percent of adults above the age of 20 are either overweight or obese. More than 64 million people in the United States have been diagnosed with one or more types of cardiovascular disease. Millions of people suffer from type 2 diabetes, high cholesterol, osteoporosis, and many other serious health conditions. While juicing may not be enough to "cure" all of these diseases, a wealth of scientific research data suggests that it does help reduce the severity or reverse the symptoms of many chronic illnesses.

Some of the so-called "diseases of civilization" include:

- Acid reflux
- Acne
- Allergies
- Alzheimer's disease
- Anemia
- Anorexia
- Arteriosclerosis
- Arthritis
- Asthma
- Auto-immune
- disorders
- Cancer
- Cardiovascular disease
- Celiac disease
- Cirrhosis (liver disease)
- Colitis
- Constipation
- Crohn's disease
- Depression
- Diabetes
- Eczema
- Gout
- Halitosis
- High cholesterol
- Hypertension
- Hypoglycemia
- Migraines
- Obesity
- Osteoporosis
- Psoriasis
- Stroke
- Thyroid problems

Explanation of Common Ailments

Acid Reflux: This condition involves failure of the lower esophageal sphincter (LES) to close completely after food passes through, which may result in stomach acid moving up into the esophagus. Common symptoms of acid reflux include chest pain (heartburn), bloating, and regurgitation. One of the most common causes for acid reflux is a hiatal hernia, though other contributing factors include obesity, eating acidic foods, smoking, and eating very large meals.

Acne: Though most commonly seen in teenagers, acne is a condition that can affect people of any age. Acne is a skin condition occurring as a result of hair follicles becoming plugged with dead skin cells and oil. Lesions may appear on the face, chest, neck, back, and shoulders—in severe cases, it can lead to permanent scarring. Factors that may trigger or exacerbate acne include hormonal changes, diet, and certain medications.

Allergies: Allergies are the body's response to a foreign substance by way of the immune system producing antibodies. The production of these antibodies can cause reactions such as inflammation of the skin, sinuses, or digestion issues. Common symptoms of allergies include congestion, runny nose, watery eyes, and hives. Some of the most common allergies are to food, insect bites, drugs, pet dander, dust, and pollen.

Alzheimer's Disease: This disease is a neurodegenerative disorder that over time, destroys memory in addition to other cognitive functions. Alzheimer's disease causes brain cells to degenerate and die, which results in progressive memory loss. There is no cure for Alzheimer's disease, and the cause is believed to be a combination of genetics, lifestyle, and environmental factors.

Anemia: Anemia is a condition involving insufficient production of red blood cells, which limits the ability of the blood to carry oxygen to your tissues. Symptoms of anemia include fatigue, pale skin, chest pain, dizziness, and cold hands or feet. Anemia can be caused by a number of factors, including iron deficiency, vitamin deficiency, bone marrow disease, or other chronic diseases.

Arteriosclerosis: Arteries are the blood vessels that carry oxygen to the heart and throughout the body. When these arteries thicken and blood flow becomes restricted, it is called arteriosclerosis. Mild cases may not produce any symptoms, but moderate to severe cases may cause leg pain, chest pain, angina, high blood pressure, and kidney failure.

Arthritis: Arthritis is a condition characterized by the inflammation of one or more joints. The symptoms of this disease include stiffness and joint pain, which often worsen with age.

Asthma: Asthma is a respiratory condition in which the airways swell and narrow, restricting breathing. There is no cure for asthma, but symptoms can be controlled with medication and lifestyle changes. Common symptoms include shortness of breath, chest tightness, wheezing, and coughing attacks. In many cases, symptoms are caused or worsened by exercise, environmental irritants, or allergies.

Cancer: There are many different types of cancer, but all share the development of abnormal cells that infiltrate and destroy bodily tissue. Symptoms vary depending on the type of cancer, as do treatments. Generally, cancer is caused by mutation of the DNA within cells—these mutations may be affected by genetics or triggered by environmental factors.

Cardiovascular Disease: A form of heart disease, cardiovascular disease typically refers to conditions involving blocked arteries, which may lead to heart attack or stroke. Common symptoms of cardiovascular disease include chest pain, shortness of breath, pain or numbness in the extremities, and abnormal heart rhythm.

Celiac Disease: Celiac disease is an autoimmune disorder exacerbated by the consumption of gluten—a protein found in wheat, barley, and rye. Symptoms of celiac disease include anemia, skin rash, fatigue, joint pain, indigestion, and acid reflux. The cause of the disease itself is unknown, but genetics are a key factor.

Cirrhosis (Liver Disease): Cirrhosis is a term used to describe the scarring left by damage to the liver as a result of various liver diseases. Damage to the liver cannot be undone, but if diagnosed early enough, it can be managed. Symptoms of cirrhosis may not appear until the damage is extensive—those symptoms may include fatigue, bleeding or bruising easily, loss of appetite, jaundice, and nausea.

Colitis: Also known as ulcerative colitis, this condition is another inflammatory bowel disease that causes long-term inflammation of the digestive tract. This condition may produce symptoms including abdominal pain, bloody stool, diarrhea, and unexplained fever.

Constipation: Constipation is a term used to describe the difficult passage of stools and a drastic decrease in the frequency of bowel movements. This condition can be treated with laxatives, and its causes are often temporary.

Crohn's Disease: Crohn's disease is a type of bowel disease caused by the inflammation of the digestive tract. This can lead to abdominal pain, diarrhea, and malnutrition. The exact cause of Crohn's is unknown, and there is no cure. The condition can be managed, however, by following a healthy diet and other therapies.

Depression: Depression is a type of mental illness characterized by persistent feelings of sadness and/or loss of interest. The condition may also produce physical symptoms, such as crying spells, irritability, fatigue, back pain, and headaches. The exact cause of depression is unknown, but risk factors may include hormone imbalance, genetics, tragedy, or trauma.

Diabetes: Also called diabetes mellitus, this is a group of diseases affecting the body's use of glucose. Symptoms of diabetes vary depending how high blood glucose levels are, but common symptoms include increased thirst, extreme hunger, frequent urination, fatigue, blurred vision, and slow-healing sores. The cause of diabetes is the decreased or halted production of insulin.

Eczema: Also called atopic dermatitis, eczema is a skin condition characterized by itchy inflammation. Eczema is a long-lasting disease that can affect the skin anywhere on the body, although the skin on the arms and behind the knees are the areas most commonly affected. Factors that may worsen eczema include smoking, stress, dry skin, dust, commercial cleaners, certain foods, and low humidity.

Gout: Gout is a complex form of arthritis that is characterized by a sudden attack of pain, swelling, and tenderness in joints. It most often affects the joint at the base of the big toe. Gout occurs as a result of the accumulation of urate crystals in the joint.

Halitosis: Also known as bad breath, halitosis may be caused by a number of things. Certain foods cause bad breath due to an increase of bacteria in your mouth. Poor dental hygiene may also contribute. Other common causes of halitosis include infections, medical conditions, or side effects from medications.

High Cholesterol: Cholesterol is the waxy substance found in lipids in blood cells. It is necessary for building healthy cells, but when your blood cholesterol levels become too high, you're at risk for serious health conditions, including heart disease. High cholesterol can only be diagnosed by a blood test, and contributing factors for the disease include inactivity, unhealthy diet, and obesity.

Hypoglycemia: Hypoglycemia is a condition in which the body produces an abnormally low level of blood sugar. This sugar is called glucose, and it is your body's main source of energy. Symptoms of hypoglycemia include confusion, sweating, anxiety, hunger, and in extreme cases, seizures. Common causes for this condition include poor diet, side effects of medications, and excessive alcohol consumption.

Migraines: A migraine is an intense headache that can cause a throbbing or pulsing sensation in the head that is often accompanied by nausea, vomiting, and photosensitivity. Though the cause of migraines is not fully known, contributing factors may include genetics and environmental factors. Migraines may also be triggered by hormonal changes, stress, medications, and certain foods.

Obesity: The term "obese" is used to describe individuals who have an excessive amount of body fat. This condition can contribute to a number of serious health problems, including heart disease, high blood pressure, and diabetes. Causes of obesity include unhealthy diet, inactivity, medical problems, and certain medications.

Osteoporosis: Osteoporosis is a condition that causes the bones to become brittle or weak, which commonly leads to fractures and breaks. Symptoms of this disease include loss of height, back pain, and frequent bone fractures. This disease is commonly the result of age, but other risk factors may include gender, race, and family history.

Psoriasis: Psoriasis is a disorder of the skin that affects the life cycle of skin cells. This condition causes the cells to accumulate quickly on the surface of the skin, resulting in a scaly appearance. These scales may be red, dry, itchy, or painful. The causes of this disease aren't fully known, and there is no cure. However, the condition can be managed with medication and other treatments.

Stroke: When the blood supply to the brain is interrupted, depriving the brain of food and oxygen, brain cells begin to die. This is referred to as a stroke. Strokes are extremely dangerous and can lead to permanent brain damage. Signs of stroke include headache, trouble walking, paralysis or numbness, and difficulty speaking. Factors known to increase stroke risk include high blood pressure, high cholesterol, and smoking.

Thyroid Problems: The thyroid is responsible for producing hormones that influence all of the body's metabolic processes. Thyroid problems vary depending on whether the disease results in the overproduction or underproduction of hormones. Overproduction of the thyroid gland is called hyperthyroidism, while underproduction is referred to as hypothyroidism.

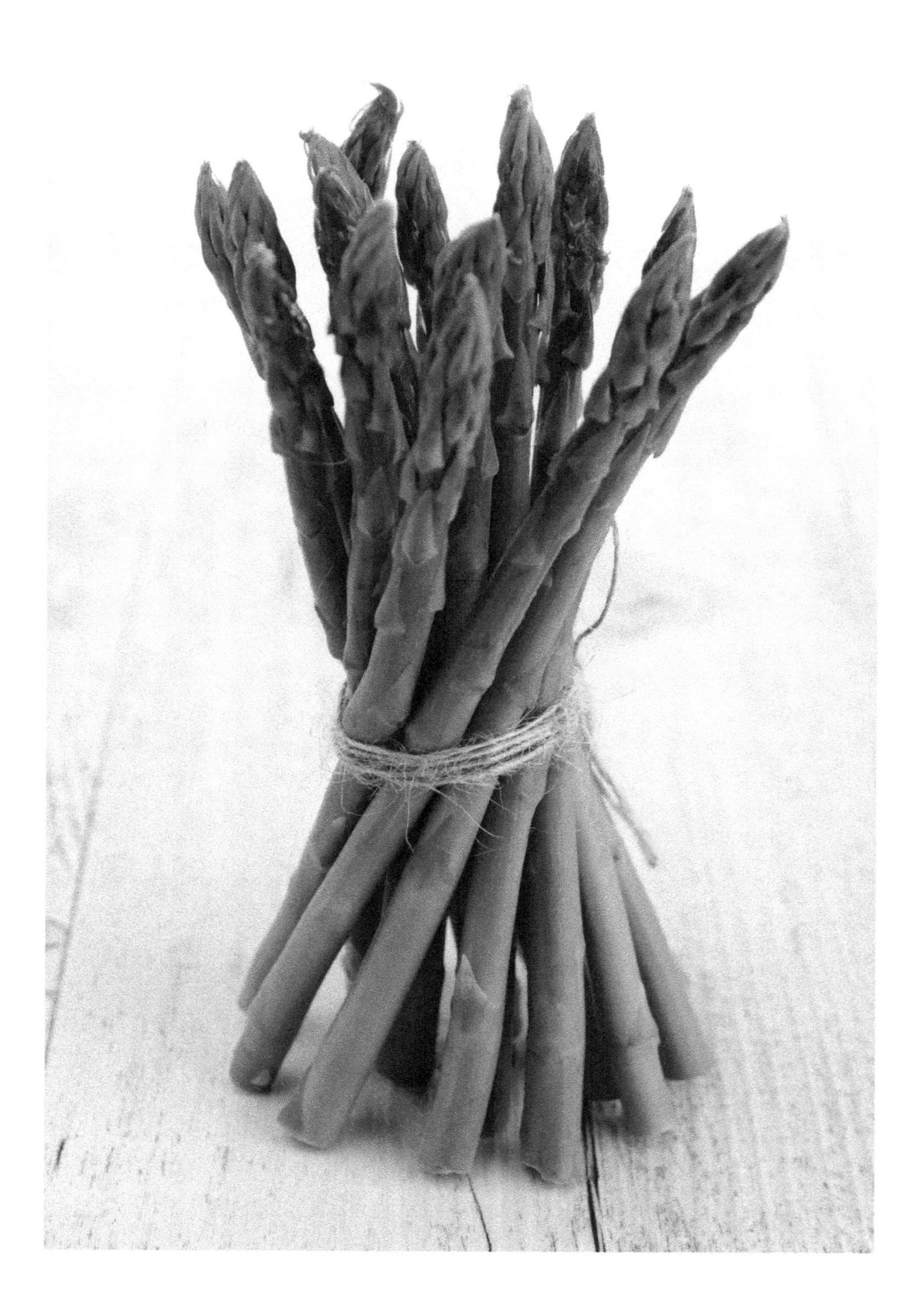

CHAPTER SIX

Juicing and Weight Loss

"A recent study, which evaluated surveys of 500 people on a living foods diet, showed amazing health benefits from choosing raw foods. (Freshly made juice is the supreme raw food.) The study showed that more than 80 percent of the people surveyed lost weight. But that was only the beginning of their transformation."

—CHERIE CALBOM

How Juicing Promotes Weight Loss

For all the great things said about juicing in this book and elsewhere, it is not a magical solution for all of your health problems—nor is it a guaranteed method of weight loss. (And there is no such thing as a "fat burning" juice or "negative calorie" foods.) Like all lifestyle changes, using juicing to promote weight loss will still require your hard work and dedication. If you are willing to put in the effort, however, juicing can certainly help you to lose weight.

There are many reasons why juicing is helpful in promoting weight loss. For one thing, replacing typical meals of processed or fast foods with freshly squeezed juice will not only provide an increase in nutrient content, but it will also offer a significant reduction in calories. The basic science of weight loss is this: if you burn more calories than you consume, you will lose weight. This doesn't mean that you have to spend two hours on the treadmill every day just to burn off the food you eat. Remember that your body burns calories throughout the day just by keeping your heart pumping and your other organs functioning.

Unfortunately, many individuals in Western culture take in way too many calories on a daily basis: much more than their bodies need to function. This results in excess calories that are not immediately needed being converted to fat and stored. If a majority of those excess calories are derived from processed or fast foods, the toxins from those foods will also be stored along with the new fat cells. Over time, your body becomes literally weighed down, and your organs may not function as well as they once did. This can lead to more weight gain, making it a self-perpetuating cycle.

The key to losing weight is to create a calorie deficit so your body has to burn stored fat for fuel. Do not misconstrue this to mean that you should only consume a few hundred calories a day—you may lose weight quickly using this method, but it will be neither healthy nor sustainable. Your body needs a certain number of calories each day just to function, and if you go below that number, it could have negative effects on your health and even halt your weight loss entirely. The minimum number of calories your body requires on a daily basis to maintain necessary functions is referred to as your basal metabolic rate (BMR).

As part of a healthy diet, juicing may help you lose weight by encouraging the flushing of excess toxins from your body, by increasing your nutrient intake, and by helping you create a calorie deficit. When you replace unhealthy, toxin-laden foods with nutrient-packed juices, you can start to restore the healthy function of your organs. Once your body is no longer being overloaded with incoming toxins, it can begin to rid itself of stored toxins. All of the nutrients in freshly pressed juices will boost your immune system and improve your organ function and overall health.

Another significant benefit of juicing for weight loss is that fruits and vegetables act as natural appetite suppressants. If you have heard about the nasty side effects associated with commercial appetite suppressants, or if you have tried them yourself, you should be thrilled to learn that the solution is much easier than you may have thought. Because fruits and vegetables are so high in dietary fiber and other nutrients, they will help to decrease your appetite and curb cravings. If you don't have to fight feeling hungry all day, you are more likely to stick to your diet plan and achieve the weight loss you desire!

Juicing as Part of a Weight-Loss Strategy

Though juicing at home is an excellent idea, it should not be your sole source of nutrition. Your body requires a balance of many nutrients in order for you to be healthy, and not all of them can be obtained through juicing. Engaging in a short-term juice cleanse or incorporating juicing into a healthy diet, however, can be perfectly fine. In addition to juicing and eating well, you can also boost your weight loss by engaging in regular exercise. As was mentioned earlier, you don't need to be obsessive about it by spending hours at the gym every day. Incorporating as little as thirty minutes of moderate exercise into your routine just three times a week can greatly boost your weight loss.

Making the Transition to Juicing

If you want your weight loss to be healthy and long-lasting, you should take the time to transition yourself into the habit of juicing. Making sudden, drastic changes to your diet could put undue stress on your digestive system and cause a number of unpleasant side effects. You may also be concerned about the cost of a juicer. As an alternative to juicing, you can use your blender to make fruit and vegetable smoothies. To turn your smoothies into juice, all you need to do is add extra liquid. Juicing with your blender is easy and it preserves more of the fiber content of the ingredients.

To transition into a juicing lifestyle, try replacing one meal a day with a glass of homemade juice. If your typical diet consists mainly of processed foods, a sudden increase in fiber content could wreak havoc on your digestive system. Replacing a single meal at a time with juice will help ease your body into the transition.

Once you've decided that juicing is something you'd like to incorporate into your life long-term, you can invest in a juicer. Then you can start keeping your refrigerator stocked with fresh produce so you will always have the supplies you need. Don't forget to check out your local farmers' markets for inexpensive, fresh produce!

Juicing Tips and Precautions

Though juicing provides many benefits, there are a few precautions you should be aware of before starting a juicing regimen:

- It is more difficult to measure the calories in liquids than in solid foods—if you aren't careful, you can consume a significant number of calories without realizing it.
- If you extend a juice cleanse or fast for more than a few days, your body may become deprived of essential nutrients. As a result, it may

slow down your metabolism, which may make weight loss more difficult in the future.

- If you do not transition gradually into a juice cleanse, you may feel deprived and have a difficult time sticking with it.
- Losing weight too quickly on a juicing regimen is unhealthy, and the weight loss you achieve is unlikely to last.
- It is always a good idea to wash your produce before you juice it, and you should also consider going completely organic. Commercial produce is often laced with pesticides and fertilizers that can be damaging to your health.
- The juice you make at home does not contain any preservatives, so its shelf life is much shorter than store-bought juices. As a result, harmful bacteria may creep into the juice if you don't consume it within a day or two.
- If you are fasting while engaging in a juicing regimen, you may experience negative side effects including headaches, dizziness, fatigue, and irritability.
- It is recommended that you consult with your doctor before beginning a juicing regimen. Certain individuals, such as those with diabetes, may experience blood-sugar imbalances if they are not careful.

Is a Juice Cleanse or Detox Right for You?

If you are intrigued by the idea of juicing for weight loss, or simply to improve your health, you also have the option to complete a juice cleanse or detox. A juice cleanse or detox typically consists of a three- to seven-day period during which the majority of your nutrition is derived from homemade juices. You've already learned about the benefits of juicing and the nutritional value of raw fruits and vegetables, but asking yourself the following questions will help you determine whether a juice cleanse or detox might be a good option for you:

- Do you often experience fatigue or feel sluggish and drained of energy?
- Do you suffer from food-related allergies?
- Do you suspect that you have a food allergy or intolerance?

- Do you frequently experience indigestion, bloating, or gas?
- Do you find that your bowel movements are irregular?
- Do you have frequent breakouts or other problems with your skin?

If you answered "yes" to one or more of these questions, a juice cleanse or detox might be a good option for you. Review the cleanse options that follow to determine which one might be best for you.

Two-Day Juice Fast

For two consecutive days, drink one 8- to 12-ounce serving of juice every two hours for a total of six juices per day. Make sure to incorporate a variety of fruits and vegetables in your juices and drink plenty of water throughout the day.

Three-Day Juice Cleanse

For three days, consume five juices per day in addition to one meal. Drink homemade juice for breakfast and lunch as well as for a snack before and after lunch. Drink your final juice before a dinner consisting of only whole fruits and vegetables.

Seven-Day Juice and Raw Food Cleanse

For seven consecutive days, consume three juices per day and fill the rest of your diet with raw or whole foods (nothing processed). Drink homemade juice for at least one meal and up to two snacks. Your other meals should be fruit- and vegetable-based with one to two servings of lean protein per day.

Fourteen-Day Cleansing Cycle

Begin with a three-day juice fast, consuming only homemade fruit and vegetable juices. Follow the fast with a three-day partial juice cleanse, eating two meals a day consisting of only whole fruits and vegetables while continuing to drink homemade juices for other meals and snacks. Complete the cycle with an eight-day period following a whole or raw foods diet. Do not consume any processed foods during this period, focusing on fresh produce as well as lean cuts of meat and fish. If, after completing the cleansing cycle, you wish to return to your "normal" diet, try to maintain a diet that is at least 50 percent raw food and limit your intake of processed foods.

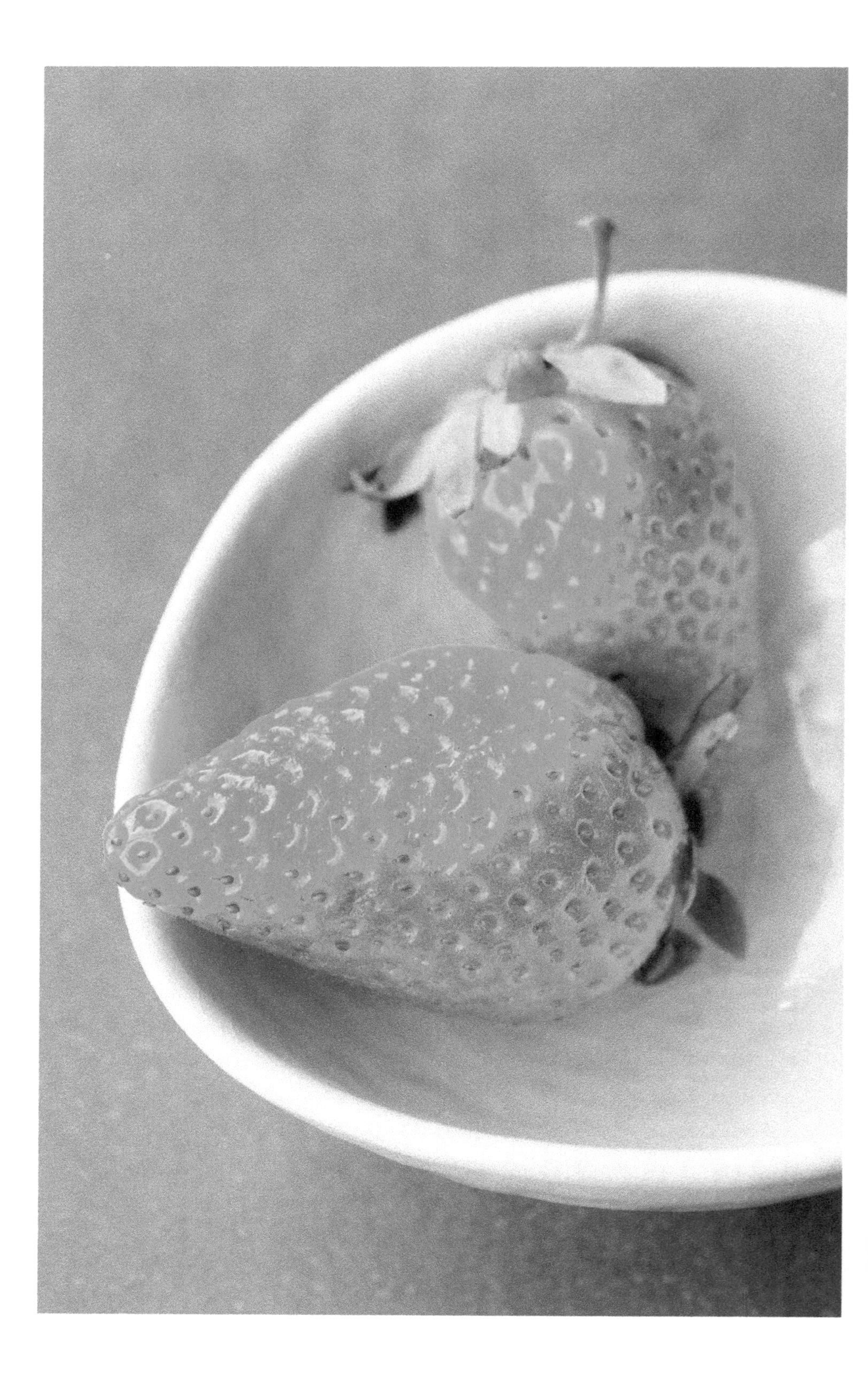

CHAPTER SEVEN

Fruit-Based Juices

"Fruit juices are a smart addition to any well-balanced diet, providing vitamins and minerals like potassium, vitamin C, and folate. Fruit juice is also a convenient way for adults and children to help reach the recommended number of daily servings of fruit and vegetables. Just one 4-ounce glass of 100-percent juice provides a full serving of fruit."

—FRUITJUICEFACTS.ORG

Health-Benefit Icons

Each juice recipe includes the top 3 benefits based on the nutritional and health information presented in Chapters 2, 3, and 4. Use the following icons as a guide.

HEALTHY DIGESTION

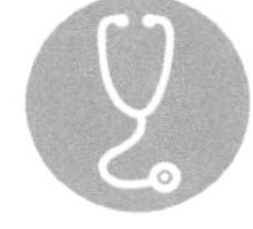

ANTI-CANCER

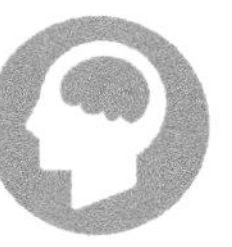

BRAIN HEALTH

HEART HEALTH

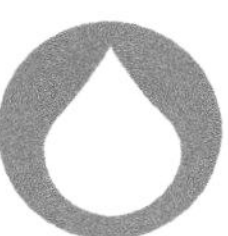

CLEANSE & DETOX

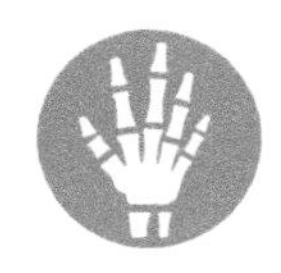

BONE & BLOOD HEALTH

Morning Melon Boost

SERVES 2

Melons such as watermelon and honeydew are an excellent source of adenosine, a chemical that helps reduce risk of stroke and cancer. Combined with the cool flavor of cantaloupe and the tang of lemon, this juice will definitely wake you up.

2 CUPS WATERMELON
2 CUPS CANTALOUPE
2 CUPS HONEYDEW
½ LEMON

1. Peel, cut, deseed, and/or chop the ingredients as needed.
2. Place a container under the juicer's spout.
3. Feed the ingredients one at a time, in the order listed, through the juicer.
4. Stir the juice and pour into glasses to serve.

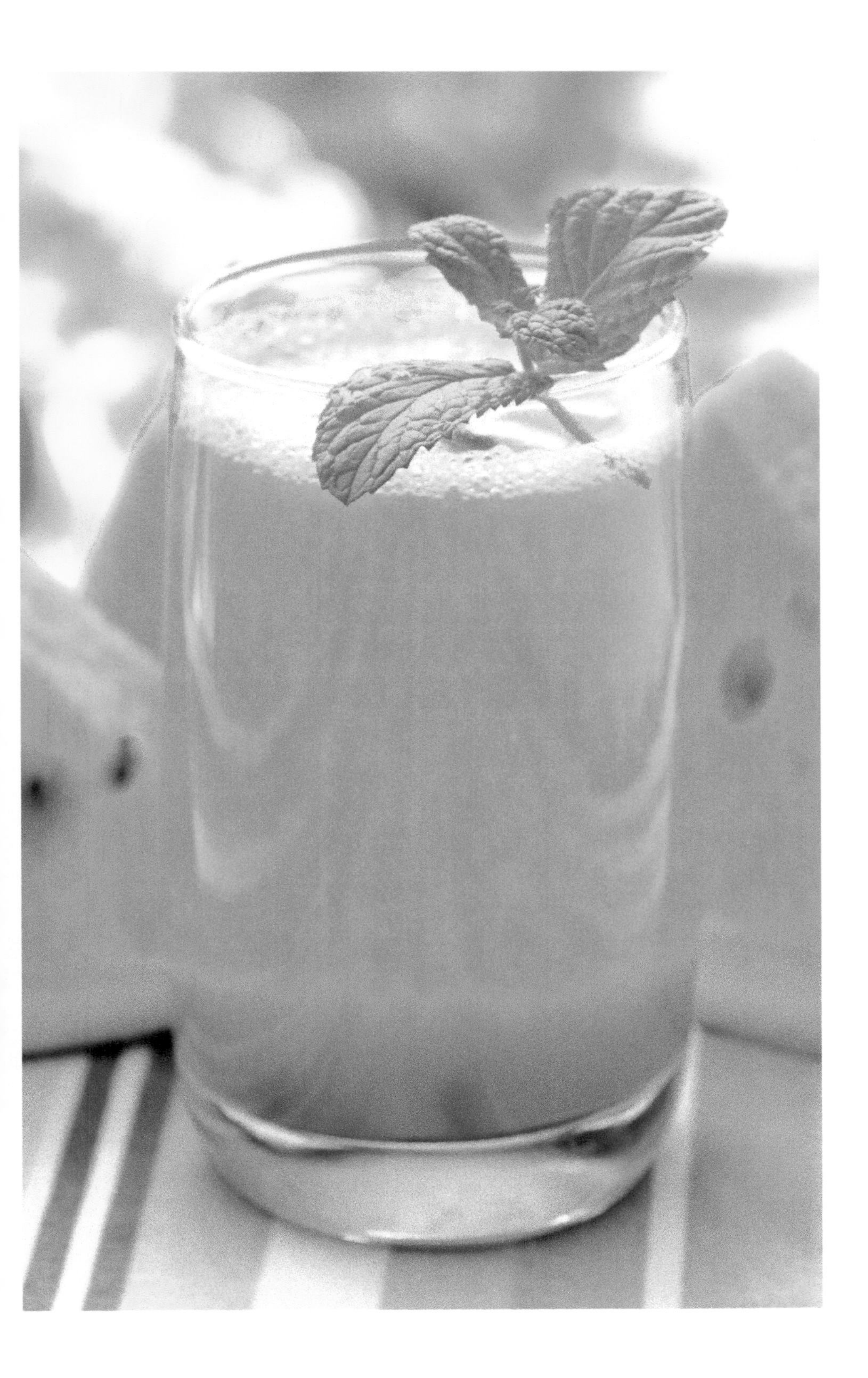

Tutti-Frutti Juice

SERVES 2

This juice is a refreshing blend of fresh fruit, sure to tickle your taste buds. In addition to its delicious flavor, this juice is full of powerful antioxidants that will help repair cellular damage caused by free radicals.

1 RIPE GRAPEFRUIT
1 CUP BLUEBERRIES
1 CUP RED GRAPES
1 SMALL APPLE

1. Peel, cut, deseed, and/or chop the ingredients as needed.
2. Place a container under the juicer's spout.
3. Feed the ingredients one at a time, in the order listed, through the juicer.
4. Stir the juice and pour into glasses to serve.

Easy Apple Celery Juice

SERVES 2

As simple as it is, this juice is surprisingly tasty. The combination of crisp apples and celery with a splash of lime juice is refreshing, rejuvenating, and incredibly good for you!

3 MEDIUM APPLES
2 MEDIUM STALKS CELERY
2 TABLESPOONS FRESHLY SQUEEZED LIME JUICE

1. Peel, cut, deseed, and/or chop the ingredients as needed.
2. Place a container under the juicer's spout.
3. Feed the apples and celery through the juicer.
4. Stir the lime juice into the juice and pour into glasses to serve.

Blueberry Beet Juice

SERVES 2

Blueberries contain flavonoids, a powerful antioxidant, as well as a type of dietary fiber called pectin. In combination with the vitamin and mineral content of beets, this juice packs a powerful nutritional punch.

2 CUPS BLUEBERRIES
2 SMALL BEETS
1 SMALL APPLE

1. Peel, cut, deseed, and/or chop the ingredients as needed.
2. Place a container under the juicer's spout.
3. Feed the ingredients one at a time, in the order listed, through the juicer.
4. Stir the juice and pour into glasses to serve.

Mango Gazpacho Juice

SERVES 2

This juice is like nothing you've ever tasted before. The unique combination of ripe mango and plum tomatoes, accented by bell pepper and a hint of cilantro, is utterly refreshing.

2 RIPE PLUM TOMATOES
1 RIPE MANGO
½ SMALL ORANGE BELL PEPPER
½ LIME
3 SPRIGS CILANTRO

1. Peel, cut, deseed, and/or chop the ingredients as needed.
2. Place a container under the juicer's spout.
3. Feed the ingredients one at a time, in the order listed, through the juicer.
4. Stir the juice and pour into glasses to serve.

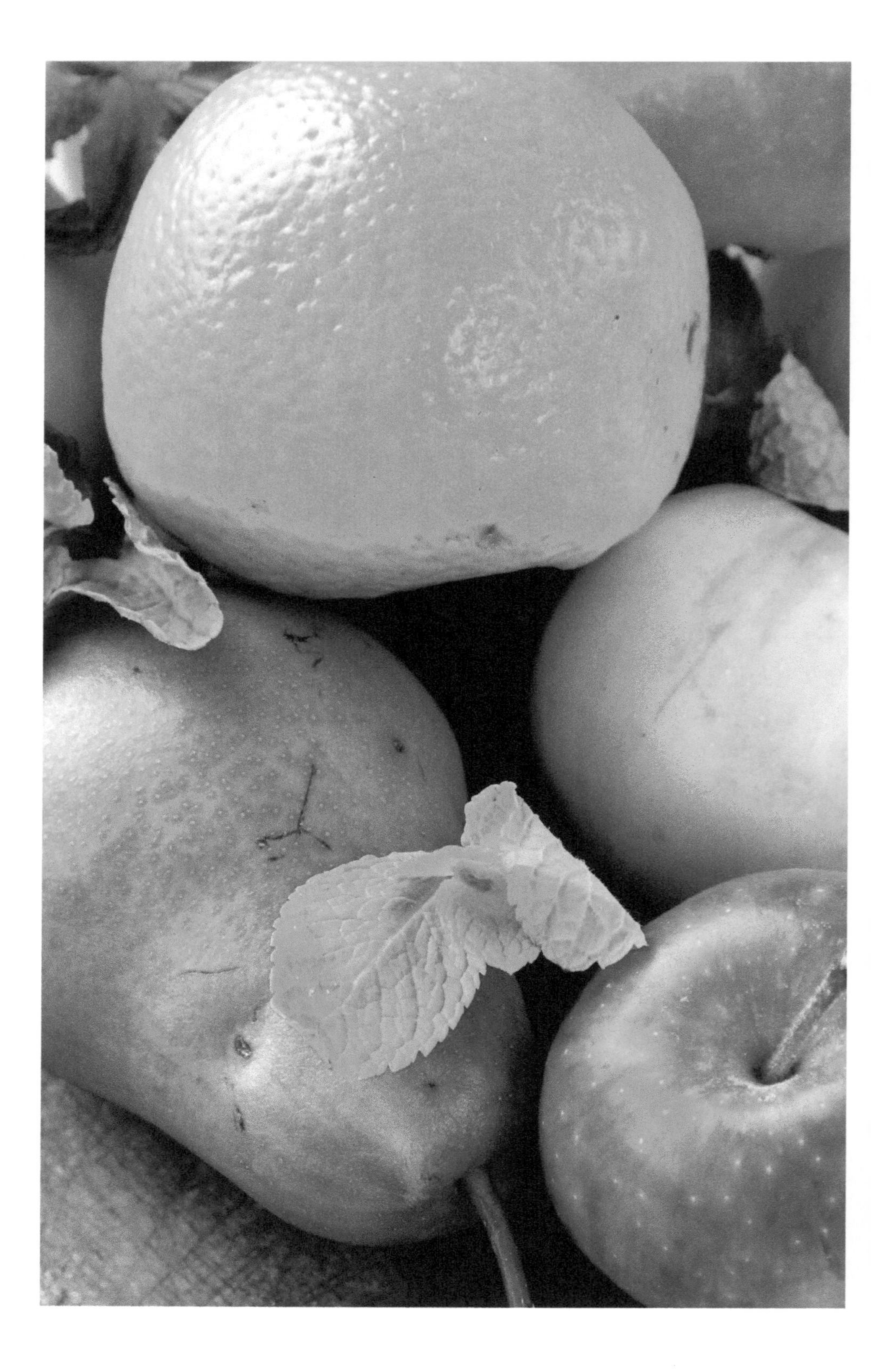

Energy Explosion Juice

SERVES 2

Loaded with vitamins and minerals, this juice is just what you need to jump-start your day. Oranges contain more than 170 different phyto-nutrients, and both apples and pears have cleansing properties that will help flush toxins from your system.

1 MEDIUM NAVEL ORANGE
1 MEDIUM APPLE
1 MEDIUM PEAR
½ BUNCH PARSLEY
½ LIME

1. Peel, cut, deseed, and/or chop the ingredients as needed.
2. Place a container under the juicer's spout.
3. Feed the ingredients one at a time, in the order listed, through the juicer.
4. Stir the juice and pour into glasses to serve.

Sparkling Kiwi Pineapple Juice

SERVES 2

No one said that fresh-pressed juice had to be boring. This fizzy fruit juice is full of healthy nutrients, and the addition of sparkling water gives it a little bit of extra class.

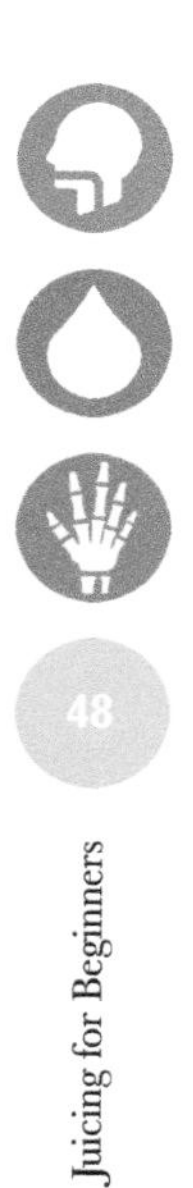

1 SMALL PINEAPPLE
3 RIPE KIWIS
1 CUP SPARKLING WATER

1. Peel, cut, deseed, and/or chop the ingredients as needed.
2. Place a container under the juicer's spout.
3. Feed the pineapple and kiwis through the juicer.
4. Stir the sparkling water into the juice and pour into glasses to serve.

Mango Melon Juice

SERVES 2

The sweet combination of mangoes and melons is enough to make you crave this incredible juice. The fact that it is loaded with antioxidants and other nutrients is just a bonus!

2 RIPE MANGOES
2 CUPS WATERMELON
1 CUP CANTALOUPE
1 TABLESPOON FRESHLY SQUEEZED LEMON JUICE

1. Peel, cut, deseed, and/or chop the ingredients as needed.
2. Place a container under the juicer's spout.
3. Feed the mangoes, watermelon, and cantaloupe through the juicer.
4. Stir the lemon juice into the juice and pour into glasses to serve.

Strawberry Lemonade Juice

SERVES 4

Juicing doesn't have to involve gulping down glasses of green liquid all day—it can be as cool and refreshing as this strawberry lemonade juice. Share it with family and friends, or keep it to yourself for a lazy day lounging by the pool.

1 CUP STRAWBERRIES
3 LEMONS
3 CUPS COLD WATER
1 TABLESPOON RAW HONEY (OPTIONAL)

1. Peel, cut, deseed, and/or chop the ingredients as needed.
2. Place a container under the juicer's spout.
3. Feed the strawberries and lemons through the juicer.
4. Stir the water and honey into the juice and pour into glasses to serve.

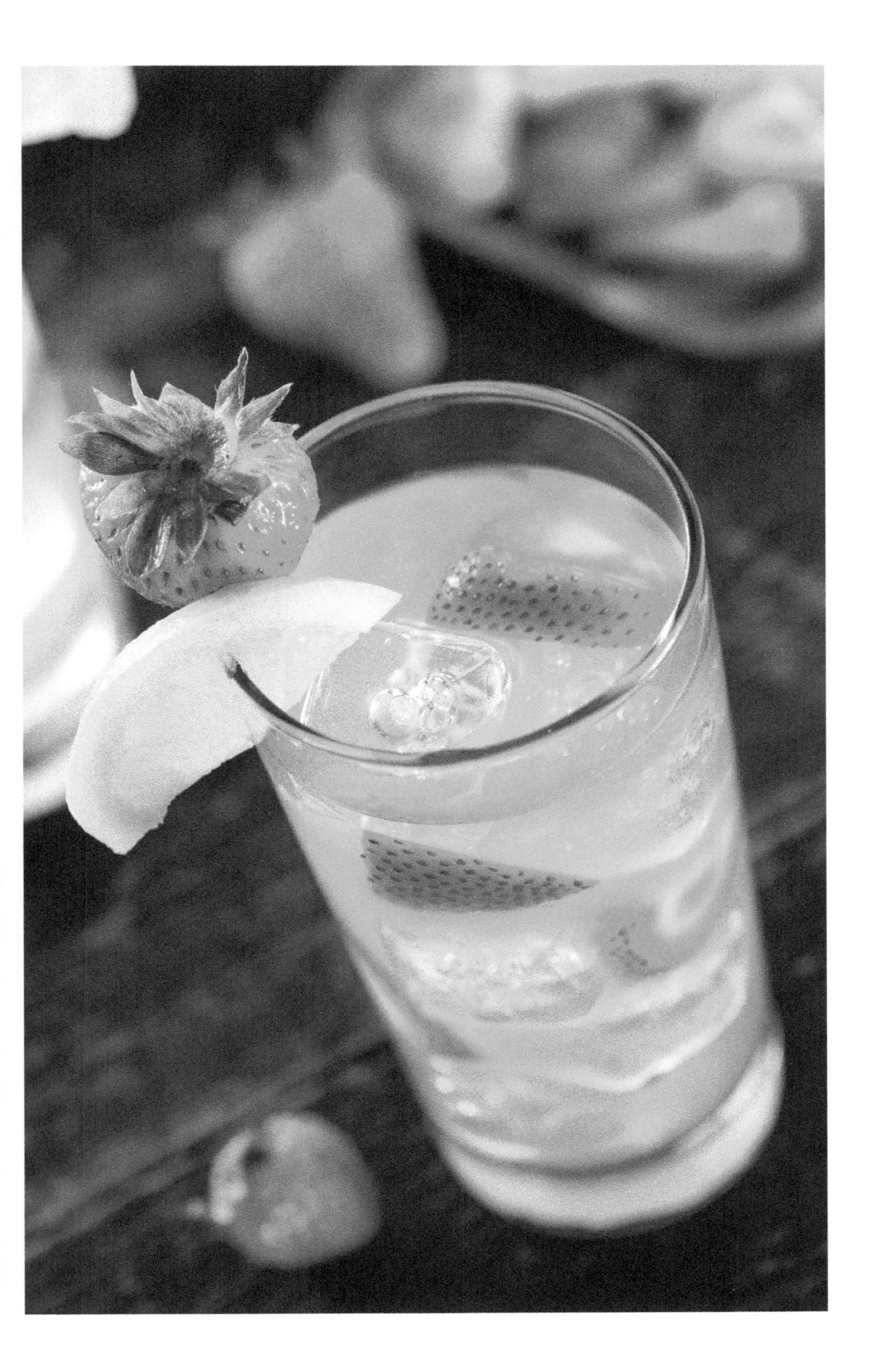

Berry Mint Blast

SERVES 2

Fresh mint helps reduce both inflammation and indigestion, and it also contains omega-3 fatty acids, which support healthy hair and skin growth. Combining mint with the fresh flavor of mixed berries makes for a juice that will leave you wanting more.

2 CUPS BLUEBERRIES
1 CUP STRAWBERRIES
1 CUP RASPBERRIES
½ CUP CURRANTS (OPTIONAL)
1 BUNCH MINT LEAVES

1. Peel, cut, deseed, and/or chop the ingredients as needed.
2. Place a container under the juicer's spout.
3. Feed the ingredients one at a time, in the order listed, through the juicer.
4. Stir the juice and pour into glasses to serve.

Cilantro Strawberry Banana Juice

SERVES 2

There is nothing quite like the taste of fresh cilantro to liven things up. Not only is this herb full of spicy flavor, it's also loaded with phyto-nutrients that help lower bad cholesterol and raise good cholesterol.

2 CUPS STRAWBERRIES
1 CUP CILANTRO
1 CUP COLD WATER
1 SMALL BANANA

1. Peel, cut, deseed, and/or chop the ingredients as needed.
2. Place a container under the juicer's spout.
3. Feed the strawberries and cilantro through the juicer.
4. In a blender, combine the water and banana and blend until smooth.
5. Add the strawberry cilantro juice and pulse to blend.
6. Pour into glasses and serve.

Blackberry Kiwi Juice Blend

SERVES 2

Kiwi is rich in vitamin C, which is essential for healing wounds and keeping teeth and gums healthy. Combined with the antioxidant power of blackberries, this juice blend is both good and good for you!

2 CUPS BLACKBERRIES
2 RIPE KIWIS
1 MEDIUM APPLE
6 SPRIGS CILANTRO

1. Peel, cut, deseed, and/or chop the ingredients as needed.
2. Place a container under the juicer's spout.
3. Feed the ingredients one at a time, in the order listed, through the juicer.
4. Stir the juice and pour into glasses to serve.

Orange-Carrot Ginger Juice

SERVES 2

The fresh flavor of orange juice in this recipe is enough to mellow out the carrot and ginger. As a result, you get all the nutritional benefits of carrots and ginger while enjoying the classic orange juice tang!

4 MEDIUM CARROTS
2 MEDIUM NAVEL ORANGES
1 SMALL APPLE
1-INCH PIECE GINGERROOT

1. Peel, cut, deseed, and/or chop the ingredients as needed.
2. Place a container under the juicer's spout.
3. Feed the ingredients one at a time, in the order listed, through the juicer.
4. Stir the juice and pour into glasses to serve.

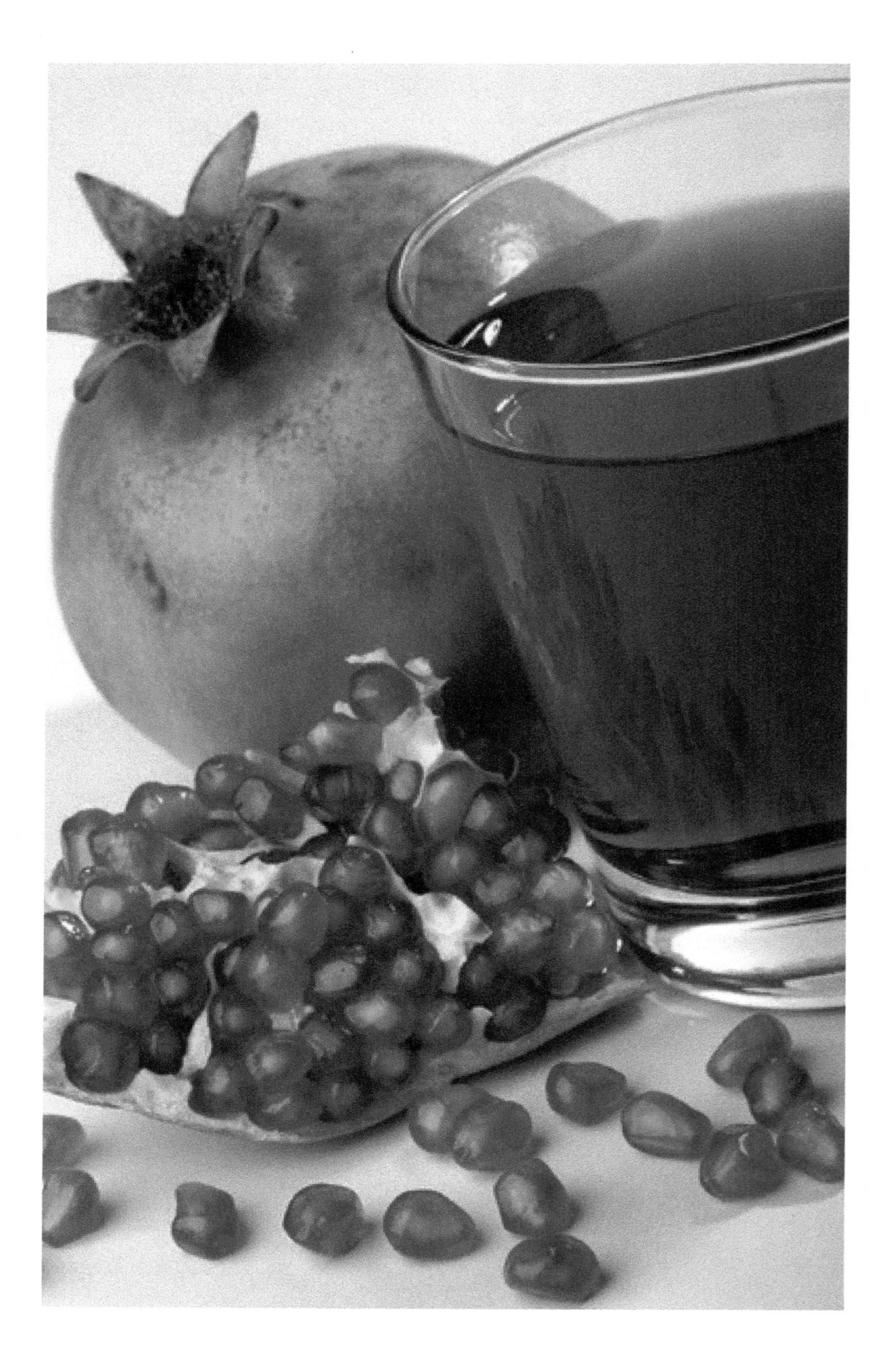

Sparkling Raspberry Pomegranate Juice

SERVES 2

This sparkling juice is unique and satisfying. If you are looking for a new and interesting recipe to shake things up, look no further!

2 CUPS RASPBERRIES
2 RIPE POMEGRANATES
1 CUP SPARKLING WATER

1. Peel and remove the seeds from the pomegranate.
2. Place a container under the juicer's spout.
3. Feed the raspberries and pomegranate seeds through the juicer.
4. Stir the sparkling water into the juice and pour into glasses to serve.

Pineapple Lavender Juice

SERVES 1

If you are looking for a unique and refreshing beverage to serve at a luncheon, or just something sweet to enjoy by yourself, this pineapple lavender juice is sure to please.

1 PINEAPPLE
1 TABLESPOON LAVENDER BLOSSOMS

1. Peel, cut, deseed, and/or chop the ingredients as needed.
2. Place a container under the juicer's spout.
3. Feed the pineapple through the juicer.
4. Using a mortar and pestle, grind the lavender blossoms into a powder.
5. Stir the lavender powder into the pineapple juice and pour into a glass to serve.

Honeydew Apple Juice

SERVES 2

If you aren't a fan of overly sweet juices, this one is just right for you. The mildness of honeydew combined with the slightly sweet flavor of apple is perfectly balanced with the crisp, refreshing kale in this juice.

2 MEDIUM APPLES
1 SMALL HONEYDEW
4 SMALL KALE LEAVES

1. Peel, cut, deseed, and/or chop the ingredients as needed.
2. Place a container under the juicer's spout.
3. Feed the ingredients one at a time, in the order listed, through the juicer.
4. Stir the juice and pour into glasses to serve.

Pretty in Pink Juice Blend

SERVES 2

This pretty pink juice is lightly sweet and full of fruit flavor. Although you may find it difficult to share, your family and friends are sure to enjoy this sweet beverage just as much as you will.

3 CUPS WATERMELON
2 CUPS RASPBERRIES
1 CUP STRAWBERRIES

1. Peel, cut, deseed, and/or chop the ingredients as needed.
2. Place a container under the juicer's spout.
3. Feed the ingredients one at a time, in the order listed, through the juicer.
4. Stir the juice and pour into glasses to serve.

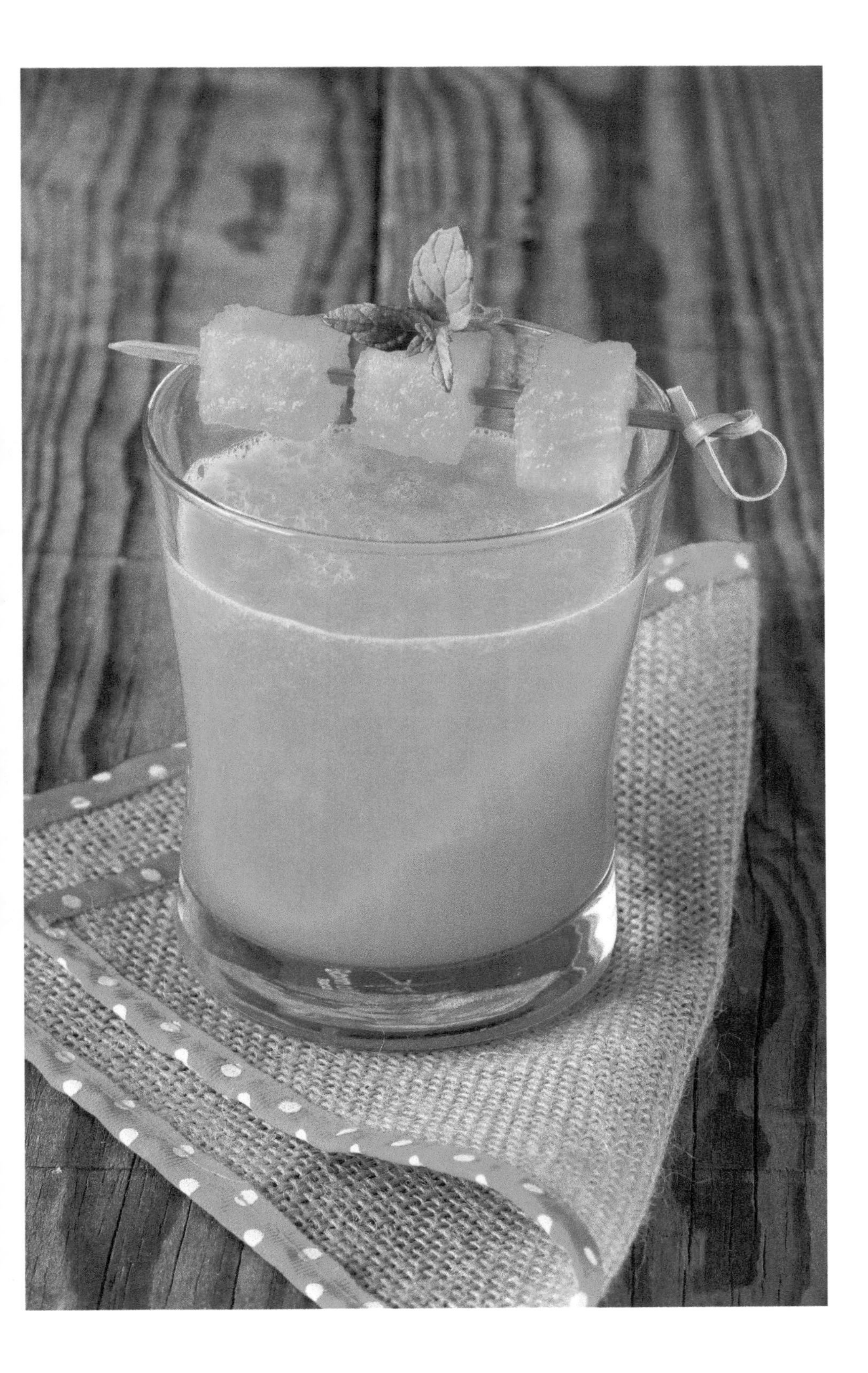

Fruity Green Juice

SERVES 2

Drinking a glass of liquid spinach may not sound appealing to you, but a glass of apple-pear-orange juice might! Using fruit juices to disguise the flavor of vegetables is both simple and delicious.

1 BUNCH SPINACH LEAVES
1 MEDIUM APPLE
1 MEDIUM PEAR
1 MEDIUM NAVEL ORANGE

1. Peel, cut, deseed, and/or chop the ingredients as needed.
2. Place a container under the juicer's spout.
3. Feed the ingredients one at a time, in the order listed, through the juicer.
4. Stir the juice and pour into glasses to serve.

Papaya Pineapple Juice Blend

SERVES 2

Pineapple contains a number of anti-inflammatory compounds, and papayas contain enzymes to promote healthy digestion. All in all, this juice will have you feeling just like new.

1 SMALL PINEAPPLE
1 PAPAYA
1 SMALL APPLE

1. Peel, cut, deseed, and/or chop the ingredients as needed.
2. Place a container under the juicer's spout.
3. Feed the ingredients one at a time, in the order listed, through the juicer.
4. Stir the juice and pour into glasses to serve.

Cucumber Melon Juice

SERVES 2

When it comes to refreshment, nothing beats this cucumber melon juice. The flavors of watermelon, cantaloupe, and honeydew blend perfectly with the water content of cucumber to create a cool, delectable beverage.

2 MEDIUM CUCUMBERS
1 CUP WATERMELON
1 CUP CANTALOUPE
1 CUP HONEYDEW

1. Peel, cut, deseed, and/or chop the ingredients as needed.
2. Place a container under the juicer's spout.
3. Feed the ingredients one at a time, in the order listed, through the juicer.
4. Stir the juice and pour into glasses to serve.

Blueberry Beauty Juice

SERVES 2

Blueberries are loaded with antioxidants. Combined with the fiber content of apples, this juice will help to flush toxins from your body, making your skin clear and your hair silky smooth.

1 ½ CUPS BLUEBERRIES
1 CUP PINEAPPLE
1 MEDIUM APPLE

1. Peel, cut, deseed, and/or chop the ingredients as needed.
2. Place a container under the juicer's spout.
3. Feed the ingredients one at a time, in the order listed, through the juicer.
4. Stir the juice and pour into glasses to serve.

Kiwi Orange Juice

SERVES 2

Oranges are known for their vitamin C content, but they also have been shown to help shrink tumors and reduce inflammation. Add the anti-aging properties of kiwi, and this juice is quite the nutritional wonder.

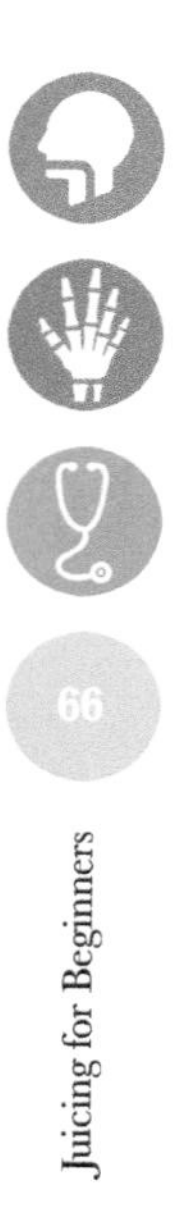

3 MEDIUM NAVEL ORANGES
3 RIPE KIWIS
1 TEASPOON LIME ZEST

1. Peel, cut, deseed, and/or chop the ingredients as needed.
2. Place a container under the juicer's spout.
3. Feed the oranges and kiwis through the juicer.
4. Stir the lime zest into the juice and pour into glasses to serve.

Mango Watermelon Juice

SERVES 2

The sweet, succulent flavor of mango blends perfectly with the mild sweetness of watermelon in this juice. In addition to its fresh fruit flavor, this juice is loaded with antioxidants.

3 CUPS WATERMELON
1 RIPE MANGO
1 TABLESPOON FRESHLY SQUEEZED LEMON JUICE

1. Peel, cut, deseed, and/or chop the ingredients as needed.
2. Place a container under the juicer's spout.
3. Feed the watermelon and mango through the juicer.
4. Stir the lemon juice into the juice and pour into glasses to serve.

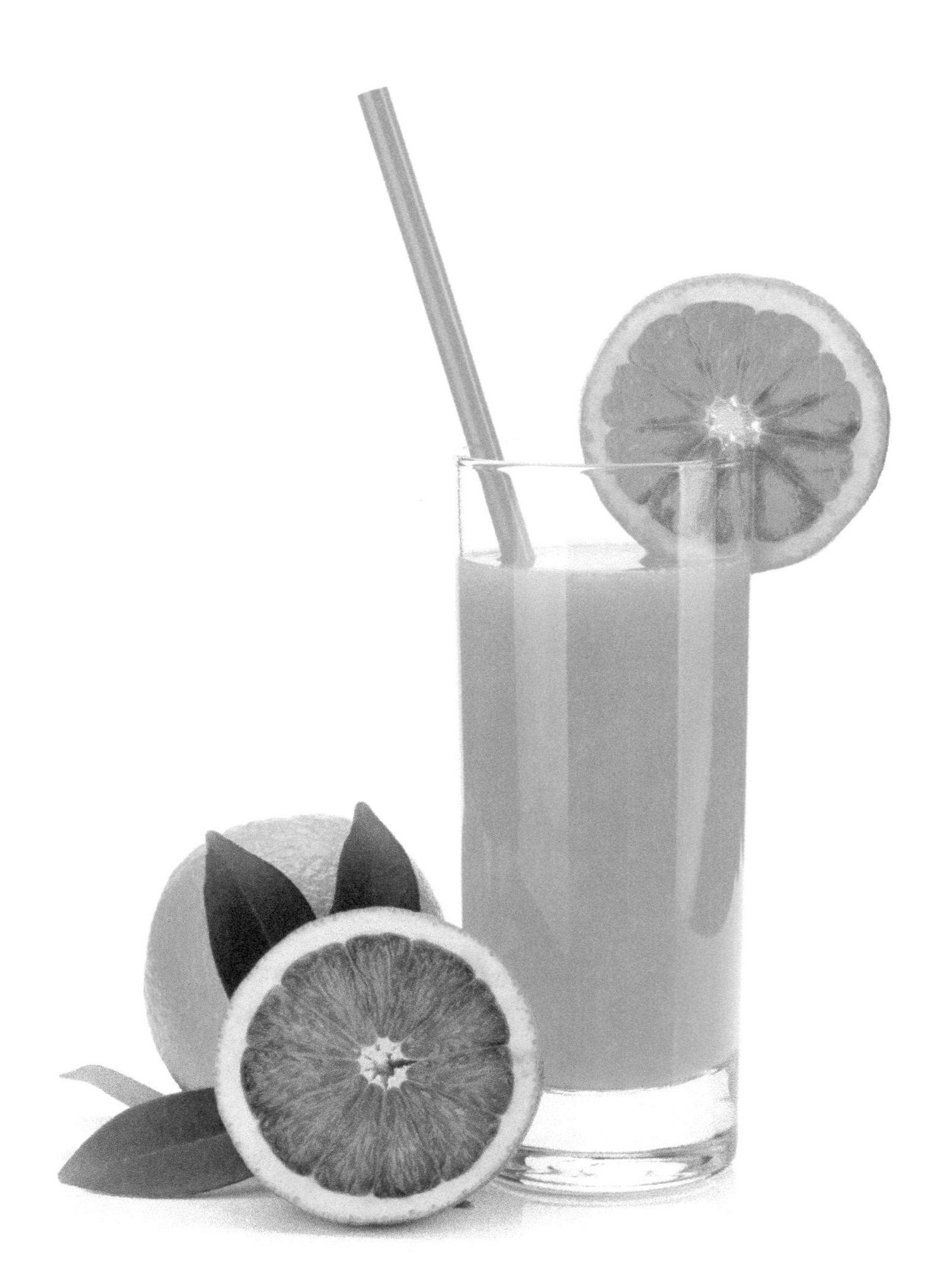

Citrus Sunrise Juice

SERVES 2

This juice is very easy to make—you don't even need a juicer! Simply juice the citrus fruits by hand and layer each juice in glasses to serve. This beverage is as beautiful as it is refreshing.

2 MEDIUM BLOOD ORANGES, HALVED
2 MEDIUM NAVEL ORANGES, HALVED
1 SMALL PINK GRAPEFRUIT, HALVED

1. Using a citrus press or hand juicer, juice the blood oranges. Divide the juice between two glasses.
2. Juice the navel oranges and divide the juice between the glasses.
3. Juice the grapefruit, divide the juice between the glasses, and serve.

Peachy Pineapple Cooler

SERVES 2

Whether you are in the mood for a sweet snack or are looking for a refreshing beverage to enjoy by the pool, this peachy pineapple cooler is the perfect drink.

2 MEDIUM PEACHES OR NECTARINES
1 SMALL PINEAPPLE
1 SMALL APPLE
½ CUP SPARKLING WATER

1. Peel, cut, deseed, and/or chop the ingredients as needed.
2. Place a container under the juicer's spout.
3. Feed the peaches, pineapple, and apple through the juicer.
4. Stir the sparkling water into the juice and pour into glasses to serve.

Watermelon Gazpacho Juice

SERVES 2

Watermelon gazpacho is a cool summer soup made from watermelon and cucumber. This recipe combines all of the delicious and healthy ingredients of watermelon gazpacho into a sippable beverage.

3 CUPS WATERMELON
1 CUP CUCUMBER
1 TABLESPOON FRESHLY SQUEEZED LIME JUICE

1. Peel, cut, deseed, and/or chop the ingredients as needed.
2. Place a container under the juicer's spout.
3. Feed the watermelon and cucumber through the juicer.
4. Stir the lime juice into the juice and pour into glasses to serve.

Coconut Cabana Juice

SERVES 2

Sweet and simple, this juice is just what you need to slake your thirst. Coconut water is rich in electrolytes and other ingredients that ensure proper hydration. Combined with the sweetness of pineapple and a hint of lime, this coconut cabana juice is perfect!

1 CUP PINEAPPLE
½ LIME
2 CUPS COCONUT WATER

1. Peel, cut, deseed, and/or chop the ingredients as needed.
2. Place a container under the juicer's spout.
3. Feed the pineapple and lime through the juicer.
4. Stir the coconut water into the juice and pour into glasses to serve.

Razzle Dazzle Berry Juice

SERVES 2

Strawberries are known to have antiviral, anti-cancer, and antioxidant properties. Factor in their vitamin C content, and that makes these berries an incredibly healthy ingredient well suited to this dazzling berry juice.

2 CUPS BLACKBERRIES OR RASPBERRIES
1 CUP BLUEBERRIES
1 CUP STRAWBERRIES
½ CUP COLD WATER
1 TABLESPOON ORANGE ZEST

1. Place a container under the juicer's spout.
2. Feed the berries through the juicer.
3. Stir the water and orange zest into the juice and pour into glasses to serve.

Tropical Fruit Juice Blend

SERVES 2

Pineapple is an excellent source of vitamin C, iron, and potassium. It also contains bromelain and other anti-inflammatory compounds that help to promote joint health.

1 RIPE MANGO
1 MEDIUM ORANGE
½ PINEAPPLE
1 BANANA

1. Peel, cut, deseed, and/or chop the ingredients as needed.
2. Place a container under the juicer's spout.
3. Feed the mango, orange, and pineapple through the juicer.
4. In a blender, blend the banana until smooth.
5. Stir the pureed banana into the juice and pour into glasses to serve.

Melon Agua Fresca

SERVES 2

This cool, refreshing beverage simply can't be beat. Not only is it sure to satisfy your thirst, but the melons in this recipe will provide the added bonus of both anti-cancer and antioxidant properties.

½ SMALL CANTALOUPE
½ SMALL HONEYDEW
½ LIME
1½ CUPS COLD WATER

1. Peel, cut, deseed, and/or chop the ingredients as needed.
2. Place a container under the juicer's spout.
3. Feed the cantaloupe, honeydew, and lime through the juicer.
4. Stir the water into the juice and pour into glasses to serve.

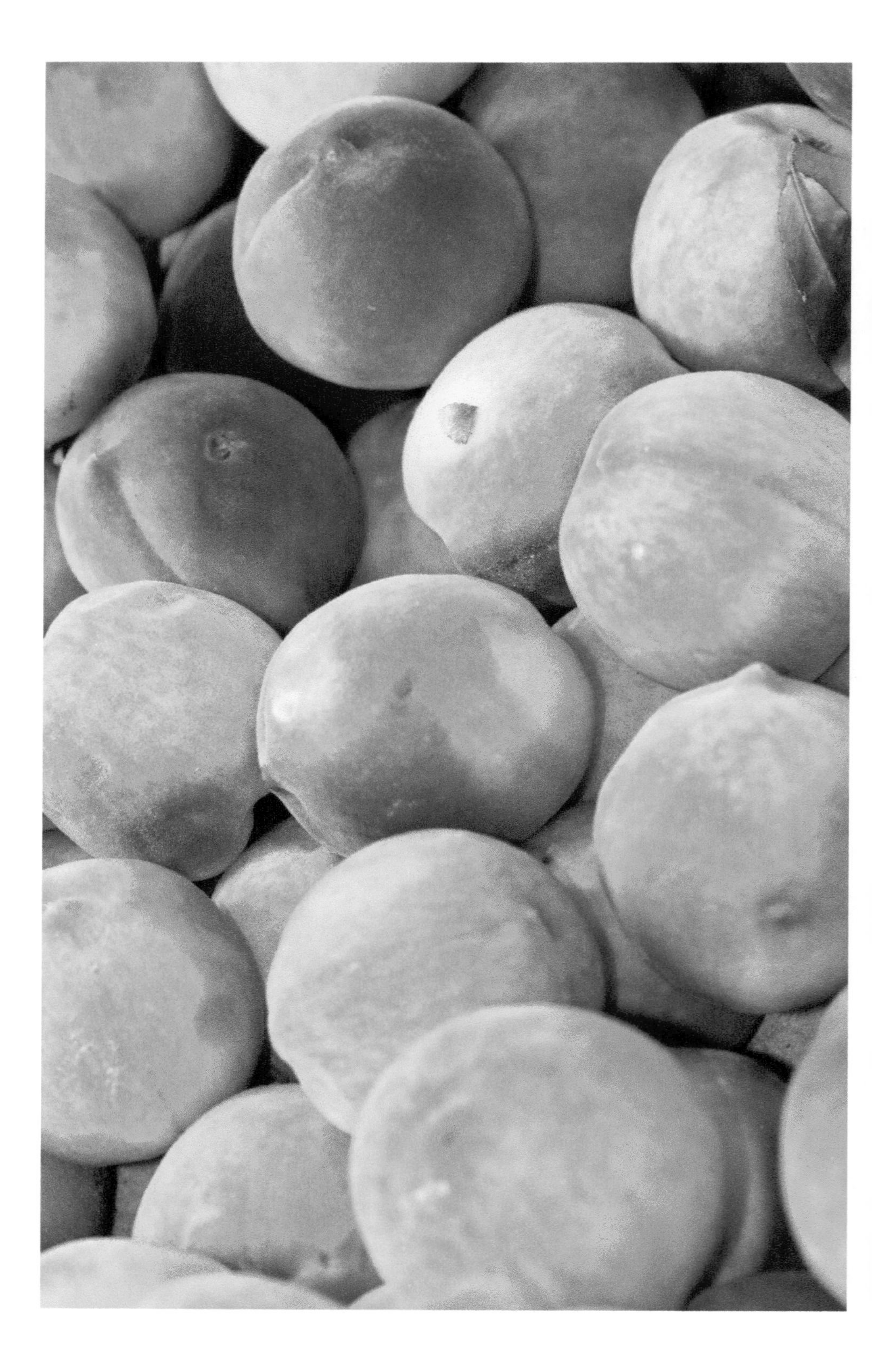

Purple Peach Parsley Juice

SERVES 2

This refreshing juice blend is just what you need to cool down on a hot day. It also makes a wonderful breakfast drink—sure to keep you fueled and focused throughout the morning.

2 MEDIUM PEACHES
1 MEDIUM APPLE
1 CUP BLUEBERRIES
1 CUP PARSLEY LEAVES

1. Peel, cut, deseed, and/or chop the ingredients as needed.
2. Place a container under the juicer's spout.
3. Feed the ingredients one at a time, in the order listed, through the juicer.
4. Stir the juice and pour into glasses to serve.

Jicama Pear Juice

SERVES 2

Jicama is a type of root vegetable known for its fiber content. In combination with carrots, pear, and lemon, this wonderful ingredient makes a fortifying juice.

2 CUPS JICAMA
2 MEDIUM CARROTS
1 MEDIUM PEAR
½ LEMON
½ LIME

1. Peel, cut, deseed, and/or chop the ingredients as needed.
2. Place a container under the juicer's spout.
3. Feed the ingredients one at a time, in the order listed, through the juicer.
4. Stir the juice and pour into glasses to serve.

Raspberry Renewal Juice

SERVES 2

Like all berries, raspberries contain vitamins C, K, and E. In addition, raspberries are a good source of folate, copper, iron, and manganese. They have also been linked to reduced cholesterol and have been shown to inhibit the growth of certain types of cancer.

2 CUPS RASPBERRIES
1 LARGE CARROT
1 MEDIUM PEAR
1 TABLESPOON FRESHLY SQUEEZED LEMON JUICE

1. Peel, cut, deseed, and/or chop the ingredients as needed.
2. Place a container under the juicer's spout.
3. Feed the raspberries, carrot, and pear through the juicer.
4. Stir the lemon juice into the juice and pour into glasses to serve.

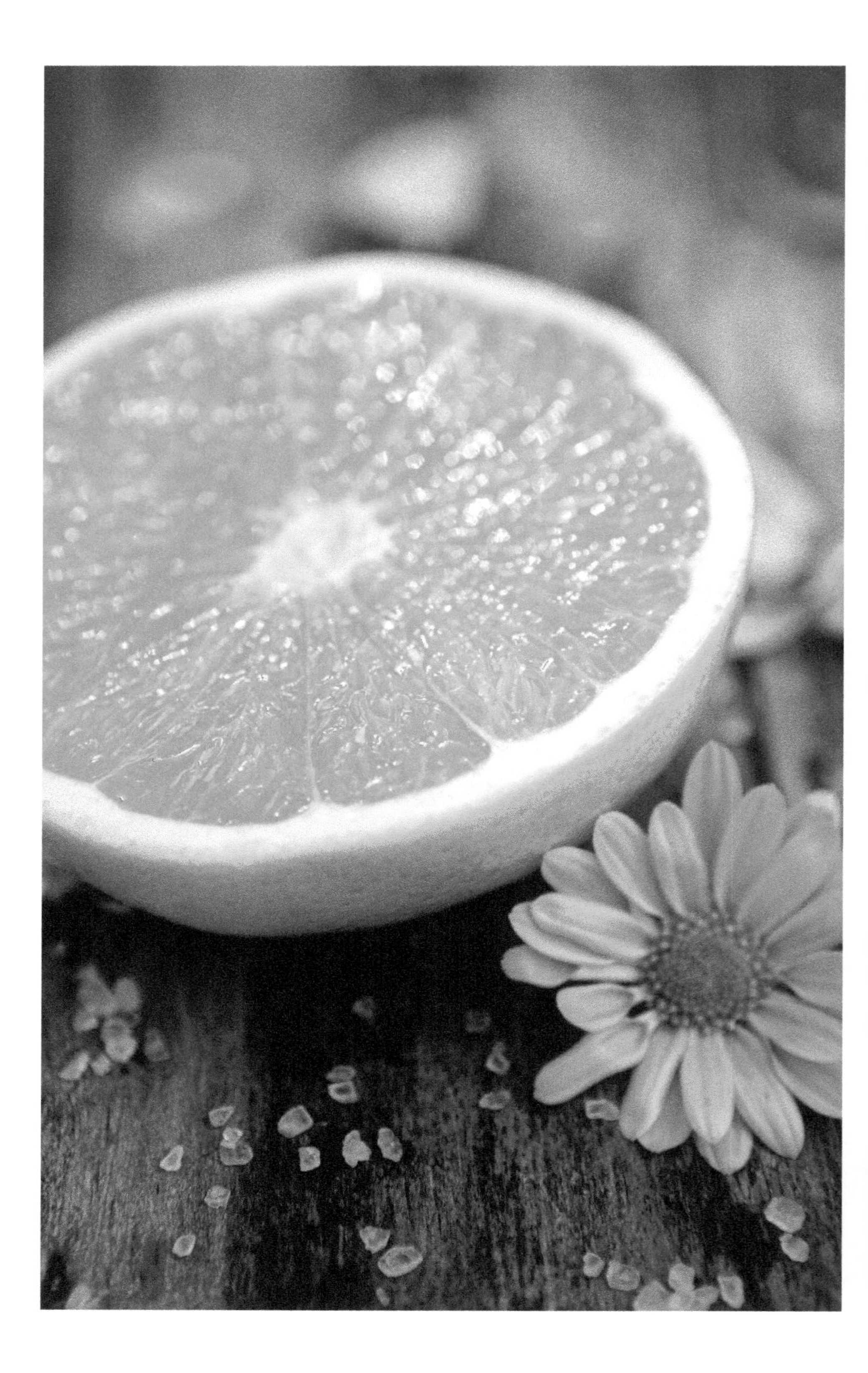

Pink Grapefruit Delight

SERVES 2

Grapefruit is rich in vitamin C like all citrus fruits, but that's not all it's good for. This fruit also contains limonene, a compound that has been shown to reduce the risk for breast cancer.

2 SMALL PINK GRAPEFRUITS
2 LIMES
1 CUP COLD WATER
1 TABLESPOON RAW HONEY (OPTIONAL)
1 TEASPOON LEMON ZEST

1. Peel, cut, deseed, and/or chop the ingredients as needed.
2. Place a container under the juicer's spout.
3. Feed the grapefruits and limes through the juicer.
4. Stir the water, honey, and lemon zest into the juice and pour into glasses to serve.

Easy Breezy Citrus Blend

SERVES 2

Citrus fruits are an excellent source of healthy vitamins and minerals. This recipe is the perfect combination of tangerine, orange, and grapefruit juice flavored with a hint of lime.

2 MEDIUM TANGERINES
1 MEDIUM NAVEL ORANGE
½ SMALL PINK GRAPEFRUIT
½ LIME
1 CUP COLD WATER

1. Peel, cut, deseed, and/or chop the ingredients as needed.
2. Place a container under the juicer's spout.
3. Feed the citrus fruits through the juicer.
4. Stir the water into the juice and pour into glasses to serve.

Apple Orchard Juice Blend

SERVES 2

There are so many different varieties of apple that it can be difficult to choose just one. But who says you have to? This recipe utilizes four different types of apple to produce a crisp and delicious juice blend.

2 MEDIUM GOLDEN DELICIOUS APPLES
1 MEDIUM GRANNY SMITH APPLE
1 MEDIUM GALA APPLE
1 MEDIUM RED DELICIOUS APPLE

1. Peel, cut, deseed, and/or chop the ingredients as needed.
2. Place a container under the juicer's spout.
3. Feed the apples through the juicer.
4. Stir the juice and pour into glasses to serve.

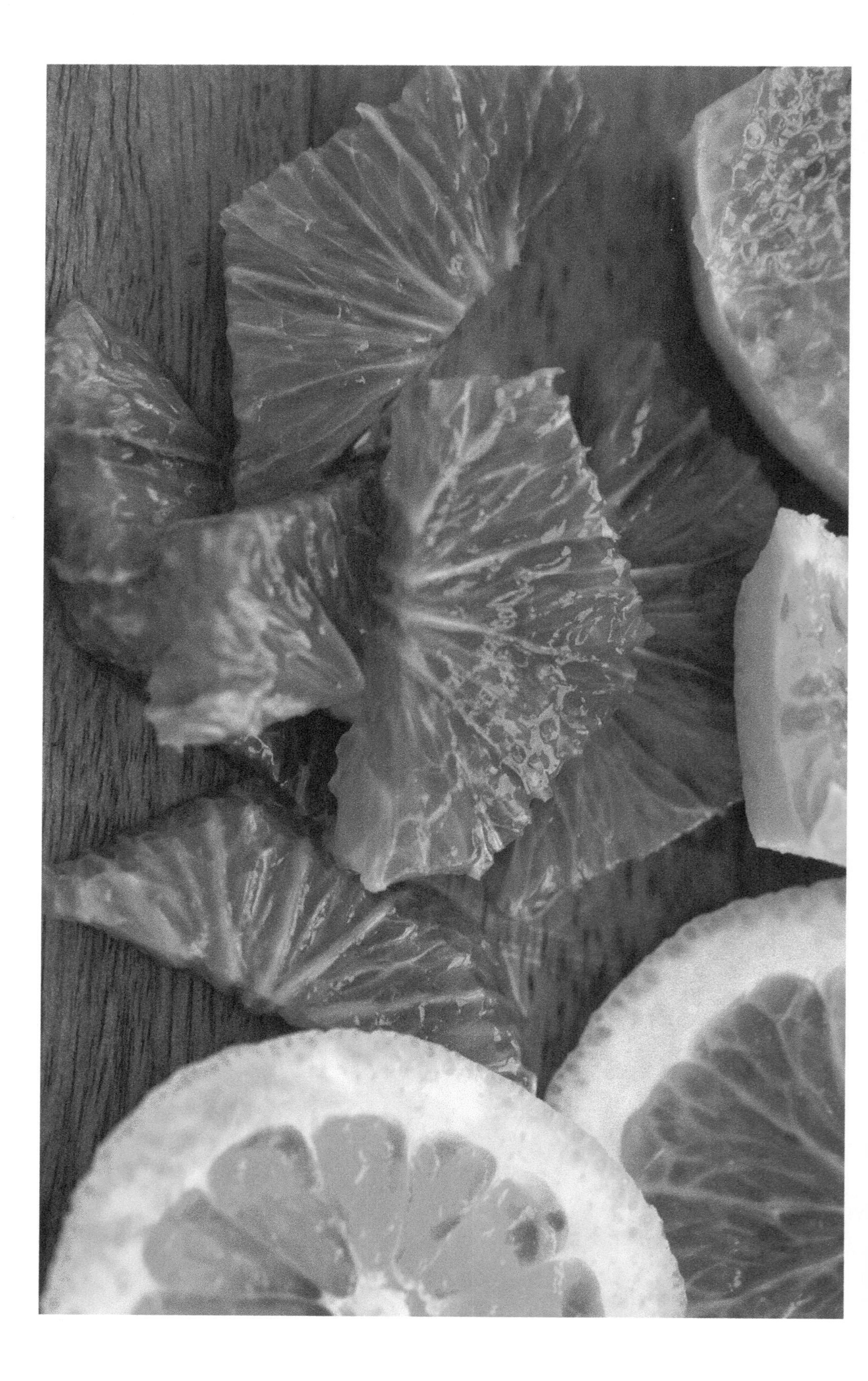

Blood Orange Bounty

SERVES 2

Blood oranges differ from traditional navel oranges in more than just color. The dark red pigment that gives the blood orange its name is the result of high levels of anthocyanins—these pigments act as an antioxidant, which makes blood oranges a better source than their orange sisters.

3 LARGE BLOOD ORANGES
2 MEDIUM APPLES
1 LARGE CARROT
1 LARGE STALK CELERY

1. Peel, cut, deseed, and/or chop the ingredients as needed.
2. Place a container under the juicer's spout.
3. Feed the ingredients one at a time, in the order listed, through the juicer.
4. Stir the juice and pour into glasses to serve.

Pear-fectly Delicious Juice

SERVES 2

Pears have been used as a natural diuretic and digestive aid for centuries. Combining them with the cool flavor and high-water content of cucumber in this recipe makes for a very refreshing beverage.

2 MEDIUM PEARS
1 SMALL CUCUMBER
1 SPRIG MINT

1. Peel, cut, deseed, and/or chop the ingredients as needed.
2. Place a container under the juicer's spout.
3. Feed the ingredients one at a time, in the order listed, through the juicer.
4. Stir the juice and pour into glasses to serve.

Banana Blackberry Juice

SERVES 2

Bananas are an excellent source of vitamin C, magnesium, and potassium, all of which help to replenish your body's stores of electrolytes. With the refreshing flavor of blackberries, this juice is the perfect post-workout drink.

2 CUPS BLACKBERRIES
1 MEDIUM APPLE
1 SMALL BANANA

1. Peel, cut, deseed, and/or chop the ingredients as needed.
2. Place a container under the juicer's spout.
3. Feed the blackberries and apple through the juicer.
4. In a blender, blend the banana until smooth.
5. Stir the pureed banana into the juice and pour into glasses to serve.

Pomegranate Peach Detox Blend

SERVES 2

Peaches are more than just a sweet, scrumptious fruit—they are also a good source of niacin (B3), which has been shown to reduce the risk for cardiovascular disease.

2 POMEGRANATES
2 MEDIUM PEACHES
1 MEDIUM NAVEL ORANGE
1 MEDIUM APPLE

1. Peel, cut, deseed, and/or chop the ingredients as needed. Remove and save the seeds from the pomegranate, while discarding the rest of the fruit.
2. Place a container under the juicer's spout.
3. Feed the ingredients one at a time, in the order listed, through the juicer.
4. Stir the juice and pour into glasses to serve.

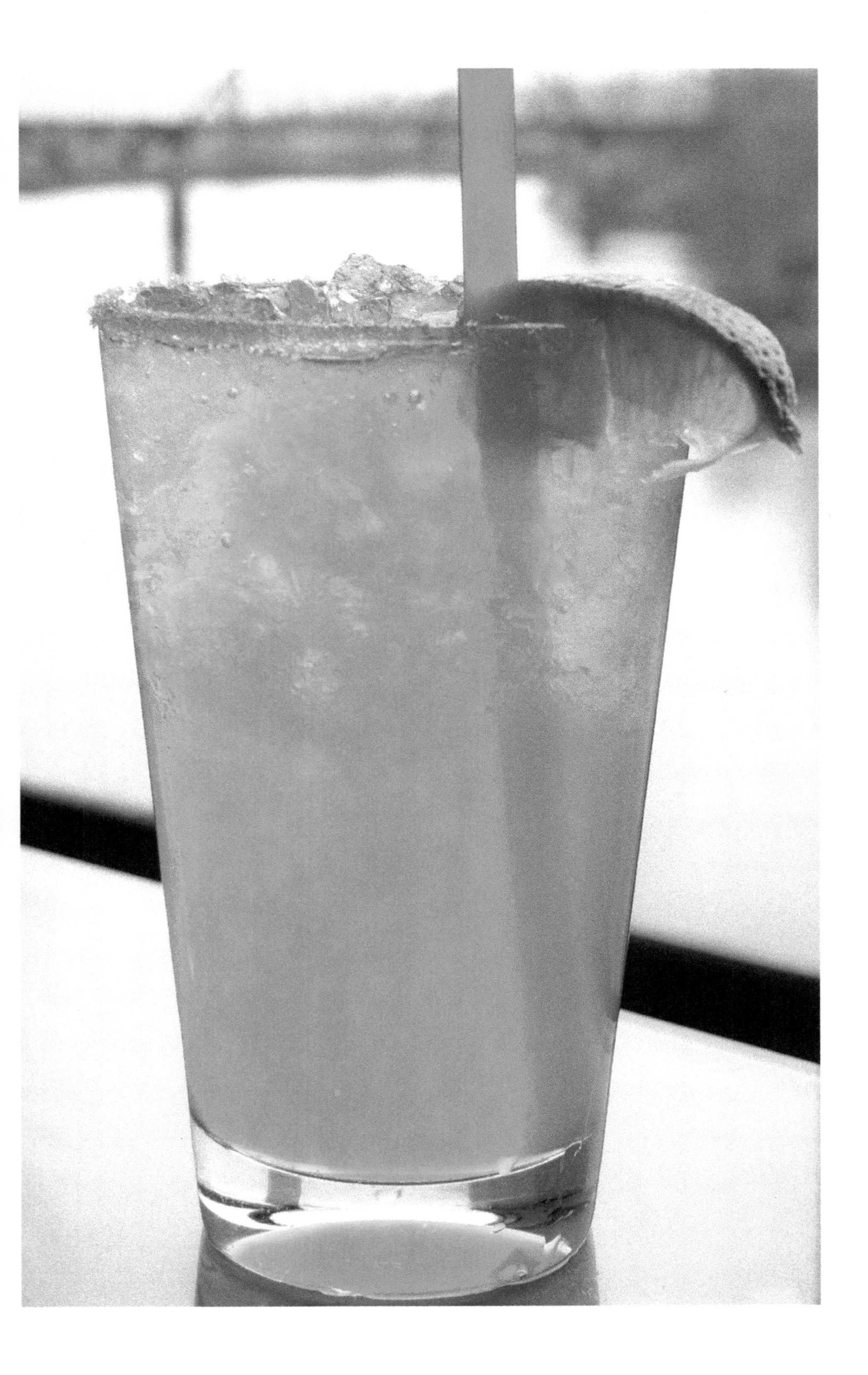

Black Cherry Almond Juice

SERVES 2

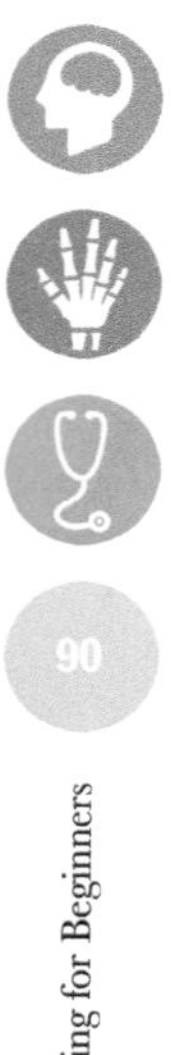

Black cherries are a good source of iron, which is essential for producing healthy blood cells. In addition, they also contain ellagic acid, a compound that has anti-cancer properties.

2 CUPS BLACK CHERRIES
2 CUPS COLD WATER
¼ CUP RAW ALMONDS

1. Peel, cut, deseed, and/or chop the ingredients as needed.
2. Place a container under the juicer's spout.
3. Feed the cherries through the juicer.
4. In a blender, combine the cherry juice, water, and almonds and blend until smooth.
5. Pour into glasses and serve.

Immunity-Boosting Blast

SERVES 2

The fruits and cilantro in this juice are full of immunity-boosting power. Packed with vitamin C, calcium, and other nutrients, these ingredients are sure to make you feel healthier and more alive.

2 MEDIUM NAVEL ORANGES
2 RIPE KIWIS
1 SMALL PINK GRAPEFRUIT
1 LEMON
6 SPRIGS CILANTRO

1. Peel, cut, deseed, and/or chop the ingredients as needed.
2. Place a container under the juicer's spout.
3. Feed the ingredients one at a time, in the order listed, through the juicer.
4. Stir the juice and pour into glasses to serve.

Passion Fruit Cocktail

SERVES 2

If you've never had passion fruit juice before, you don't know what you're missing. Not only do these fruits produce delicious juice, but they're also loaded with dietary fiber, vitamin A, and beta-carotene. This is a hand-pressed juice that doesn't require a juicer.

3 MEDIUM PASSION FRUIT, HALVED
1 MEDIUM NAVEL ORANGE, HALVED
1 CUP COLD WATER
1 TEASPOON ORANGE ZEST

1. Using a hand juicer, juice the passion fruit and pour the juice in a container.
2. Juice the orange by hand and add the juice to the container.
3. Stir the water and orange zest into the juice and pour into glasses to serve.

Lemme at 'Em Juice

SERVES 2

Lemons have been labeled as one of the most powerful fruits for detoxification—they have also been linked to cancer prevention and reduced risk for heart disease and stroke. Combining them with a variety of other nutritious ingredients makes this recipe an excellent addition to your juicing regimen.

1 ROMAINE LETTUCE HEART
2 MEDIUM GREEN APPLES
2 MEDIUM PEARS
1 LARGE CARROT
1 LARGE STALK CELERY
1 LEMON
1 LIME

1. Peel, cut, deseed, and/or chop the ingredients as needed.
2. Place a container under the juicer's spout.
3. Feed the ingredients one at a time, in the order listed, through the juicer.
4. Stir the juice and pour into glasses to serve.

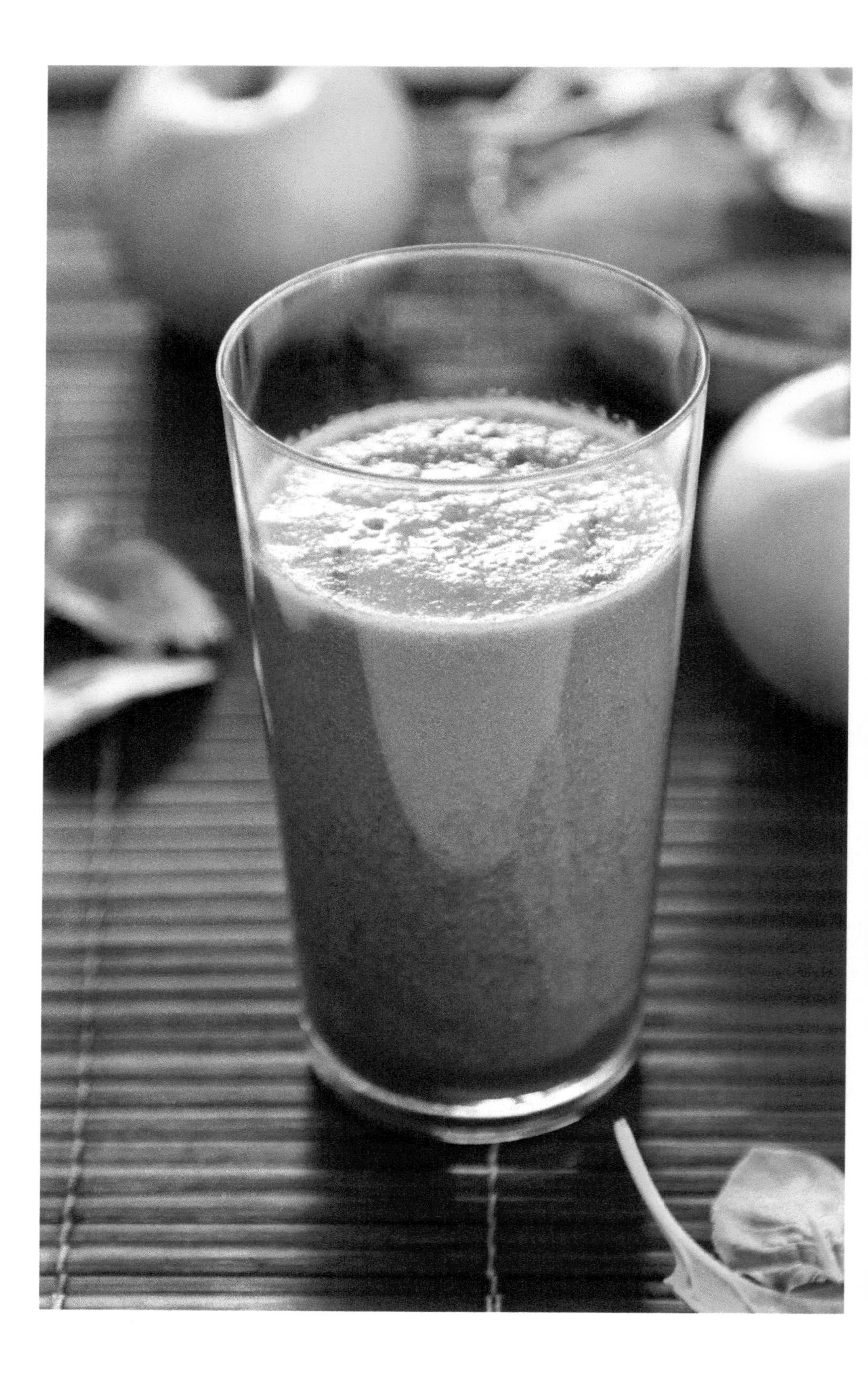

Grape Apple Punch

SERVES 2

Grapes are an excellent source of vitamins A, B, and C; they are also rich in minerals, including calcium, iron, and selenium. The antioxidants in the fruit have also been shown to have antiaging properties. This juice will do more than quench your thirst—it will kick your body into gear!

2 CUPS SEEDLESS RED GRAPES
1 MEDIUM APPLE
1 CUP KALE LEAVES
1 CUP SPINACH
½ CUP COLD WATER

1. Peel, cut, deseed, and/or chop the ingredients as needed.
2. Place a container under the juicer's spout.
3. Feed the grapes, apple, kale, and spinach through the juicer.
4. Stir the water into the juice and pour into glasses to serve.

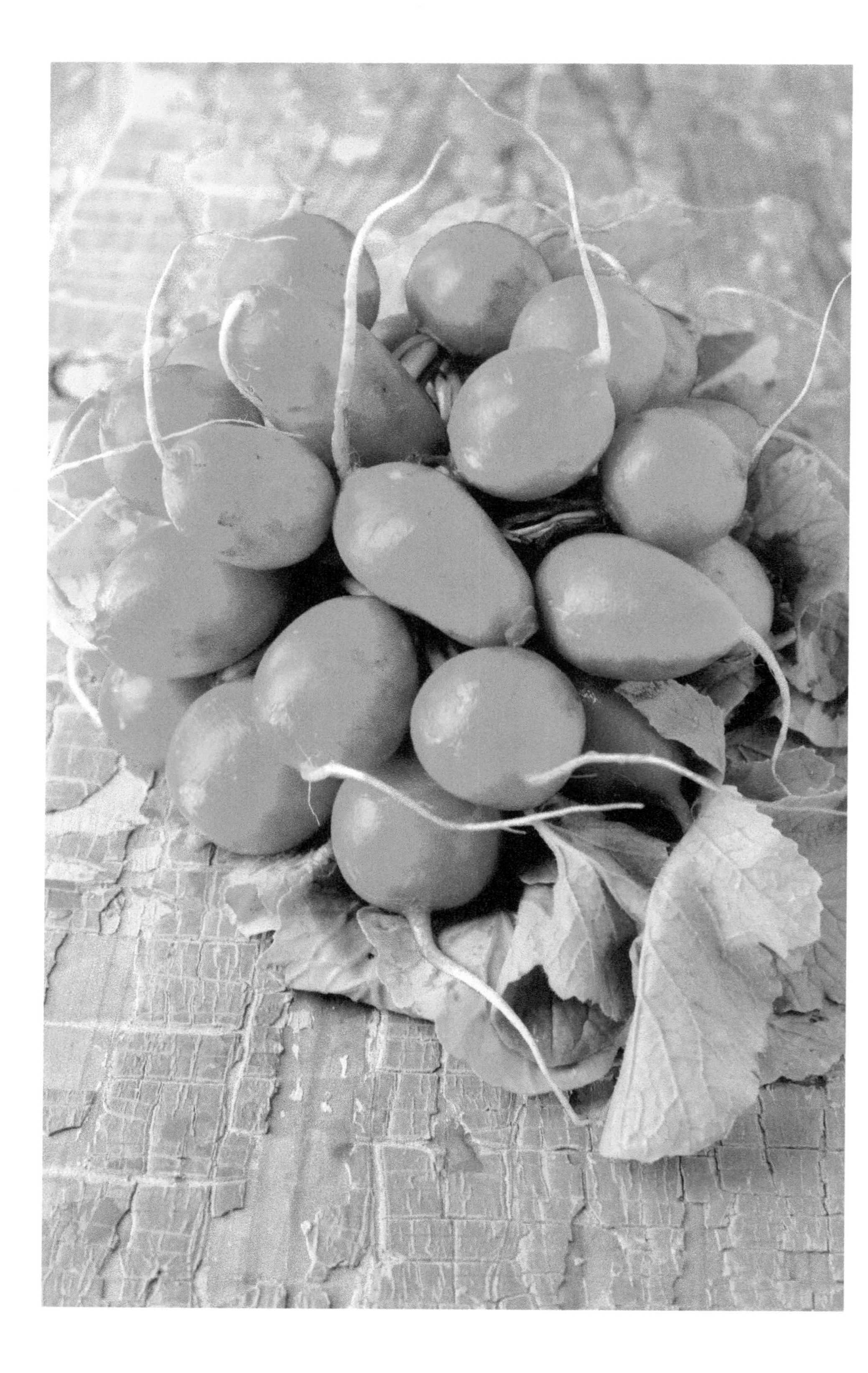

CHAPTER EIGHT

Vegetable-Based Juices

"One of the benefits of vegetables is that they have low energy density, meaning that you can eat a lot of vegetables without eating a lot of calories. This has powerful implications when it comes to weight loss—eating fewer calories while still feeling full and satisfied."

—MIKE ROUSSELL, PH.D.

Health-Benefit Icons

Each juice recipe includes the top 3 benefits based on the nutritional and health information presented in Chapters 2, 3, and 4. Use the following icons as a guide.

HEALTHY DIGESTION

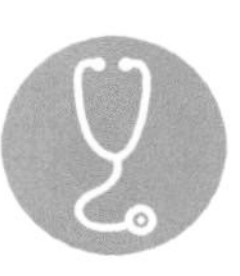

ANTI-CANCER

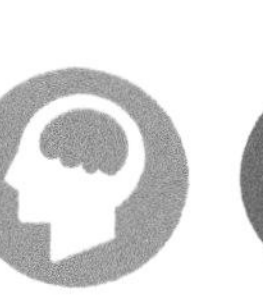

BRAIN HEALTH

HEART HEALTH

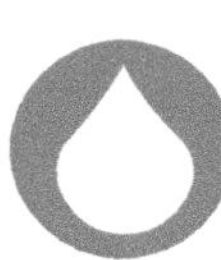

CLEANSE & DETOX

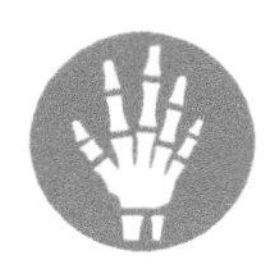

BONE & BLOOD HEALTH

Sweet Potato Power Juice

SERVES 2

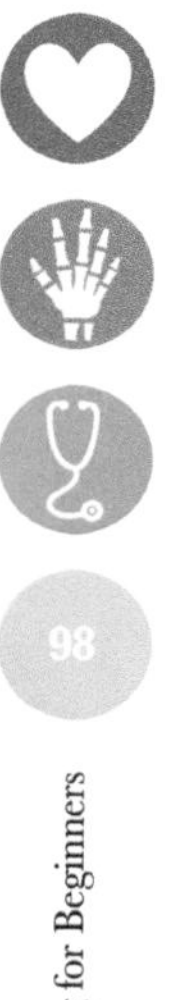

Sweet potatoes are known for their unique flavor and their benefits related to detoxification and digestive health. Sweet potatoes are also a good source of copper, iron, manganese, and magnesium.

2 MEDIUM APPLES
2 SMALL BEETS
1 LARGE SWEET POTATO
1 LARGE CARROT
1 SMALL RED BELL PEPPER

1. Peel, cut, deseed, and/or chop the ingredients as needed.
2. Place a container under the juicer's spout.
3. Feed the ingredients one at a time, in the order listed, through the juicer.
4. Stir the juice and pour into glasses to serve.

Calming Carrot Juice

SERVES 2

This carrot juice is just what you need to help you relax after a long, stressful day. The vitamins and minerals in the ingredients will help your body to recharge and refuel.

6 MEDIUM CARROTS
2 LARGE STALKS CELERY
1 SMALL ORANGE

1. Peel, cut, deseed, and/or chop the ingredients as needed.
2. Place a container under the juicer's spout.
3. Feed the ingredients one at a time, in the order listed, through the juicer.
4. Stir the juice and pour into glasses to serve.

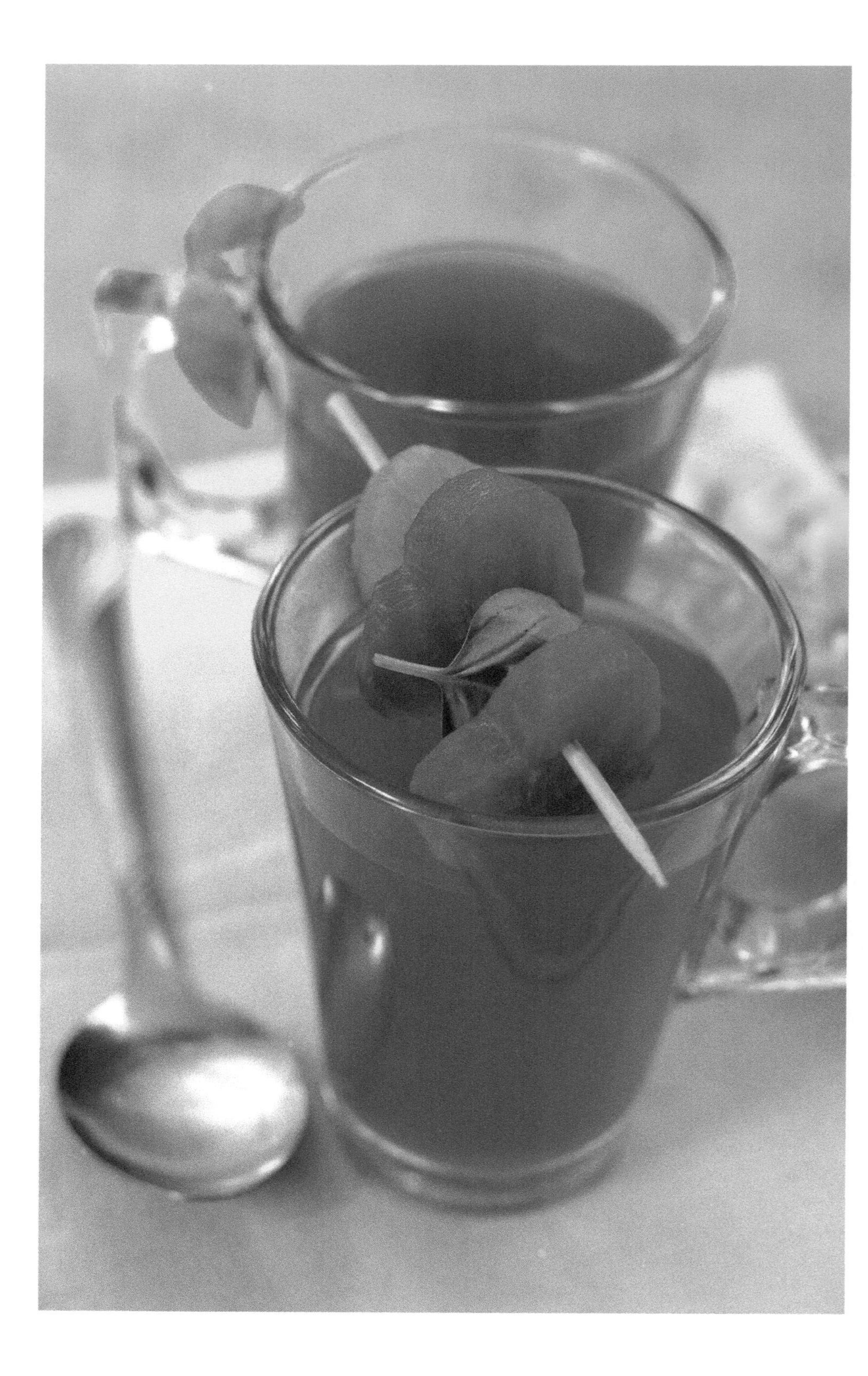

Ginger Beet Juice

SERVES 2

To make this refreshing juice, you don't even need a juicer. All you have to do is combine the ingredients in your blender and add enough water to reach the desired consistency.

2 MEDIUM BEETS
2 LARGE CARROTS
1 MEDIUM APPLE
1 CUP COLD WATER
1-INCH PIECE GINGERROOT

1. In a blender, combine all of the ingredients and blend until as smooth as possible.
2. Press the mixture through a fine mesh strainer until all of the juice is out.
3. Discard the pulp, pour into glasses, and serve.

Pick-Me-Up Juice Blend

SERVES 2

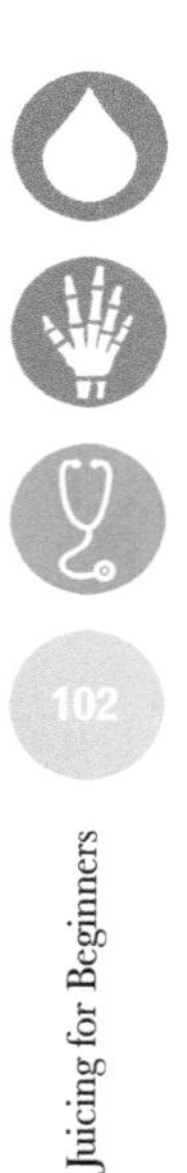

This juice blend is the perfect combination of leafy greens and bright fresh fruit. You get all of the nutritional benefits of kale, dandelion greens, and parsley, and the zesty flavor of green apple and lime.

1 MEDIUM GREEN APPLE
2 LARGE KALE LEAVES
½ BUNCH DANDELION GREENS
½ BUNCH PARSLEY LEAVES
½ LIME

1. Peel, cut, deseed, and/or chop the ingredients as needed.
2. Place a container under the juicer's spout.
3. Feed the ingredients one at a time, in the order listed, through the juicer.
4. Stir the juice and pour into glasses to serve.

Spicy Tomato Juice

SERVES 2

This spicy tomato juice may be just what you need to bring you out of a funk. Packed with nutrients and the kick of red chili, this is like nothing you've ever tried before.

6 PLUM TOMATOES
1 MEDIUM RED BELL PEPPER
1 LARGE CARROT
1 SMALL CUCUMBER
1 RED CHILI PEPPER

1. Peel, cut, deseed, and/or chop the ingredients as needed.
2. Place a container under the juicer's spout.
3. Feed the ingredients one at a time, in the order listed, through the juicer.
4. Stir the juice and pour into glasses to serve.

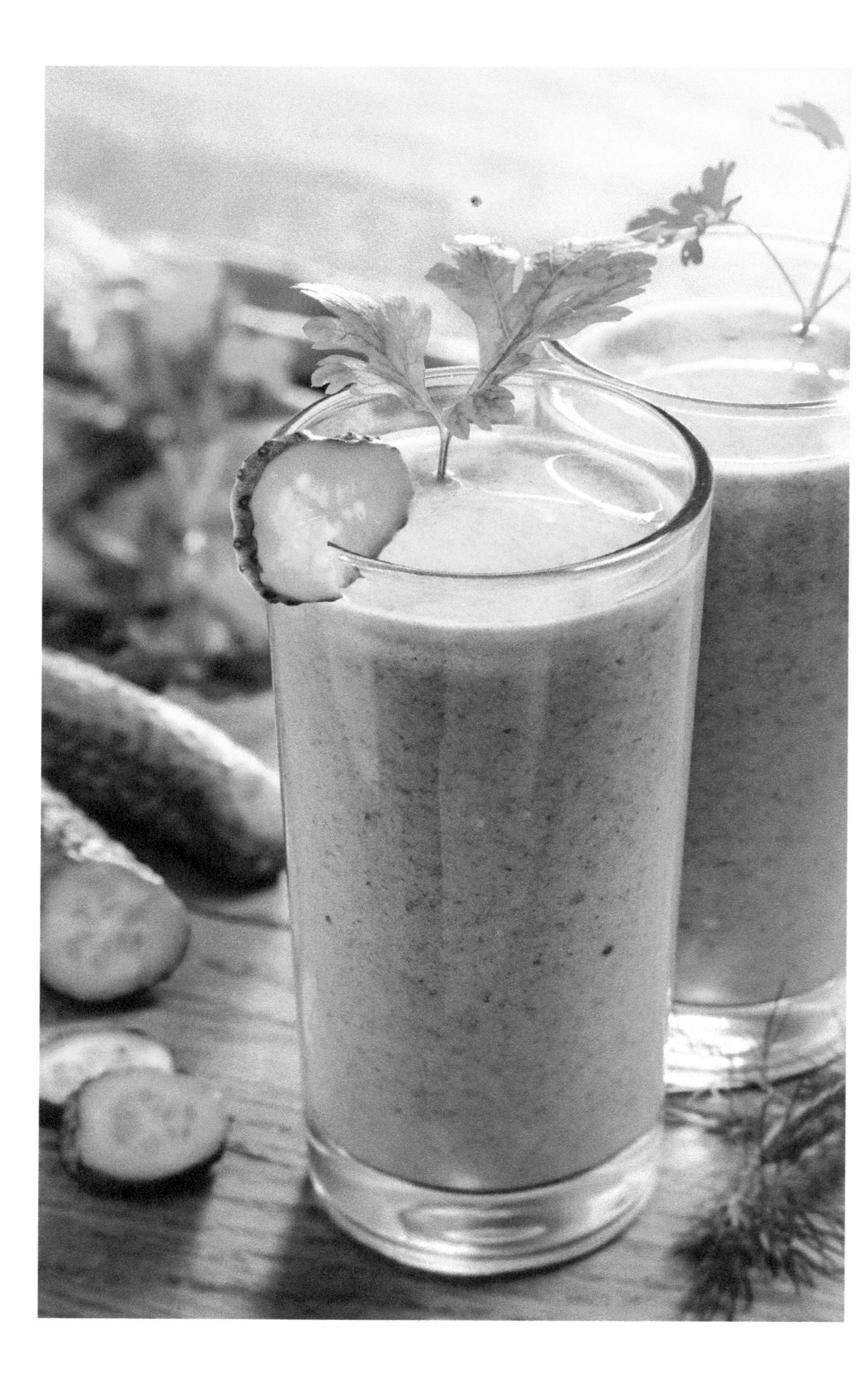

Cucumber Celery Juice

SERVES 2

This recipe is perfect for a juice cleanse or detox because it is low in calories but high in water content. In addition, both cucumber and celery are good sources of healthy nutrients, which will boost the flushing of toxins from your body.

2 LARGE STALKS CELERY
1 SMALL HEAD BROCCOLI
1 CUCUMBER
1 SMALL PEAR
½ BUNCH PARSLEY LEAVES

1. Peel, cut, deseed, and/or chop the ingredients as needed.
2. Place a container under the juicer's spout.
3. Feed the ingredients one at a time, in the order listed, through the juicer.
4. Stir the juice and pour into glasses to serve.

Rockin' Radish Juice

SERVES 2

Radishes are rich in vitamin C, folic acid, and anthocyanins, which make them valuable as a cancer-fighting food. The vegetables in this recipe also contain a combination of vitamins that help to treat skin disorders.

8 SMALL RADISHES WITH GREENS
2 CUPS BABY SPINACH LEAVES
1 LARGE CARROT
1 LARGE STALK CELERY
1 MEDIUM APPLE
½-INCH PIECE GINGERROOT

1. Peel, cut, deseed, and/or chop the ingredients as needed.
2. Place a container under the juicer's spout.
3. Feed the ingredients one at a time, in the order listed, through the juicer.
4. Stir the juice and pour into glasses to serve.

Green Machine Juice Blend

SERVES 3–4

This juice is packed with all the vitamins and minerals you need for sustenance. Not only is it incredibly nutritious, it also has a unique flavor provided by radishes and their greens.

6 RED RADISHES WITH GREENS
3 PLUM TOMATOES
2 MEDIUM BEETS
2 SMALL CARROTS
2 LARGE STALKS CELERY
2 CUPS PACKED PARSLEY LEAVES

1. Peel, cut, deseed, and/or chop the ingredients as needed.
2. Place a container under the juicer's spout.
3. Feed the ingredients one at a time, in the order listed, through the juicer.
4. Stir the juice and pour into glasses to serve.

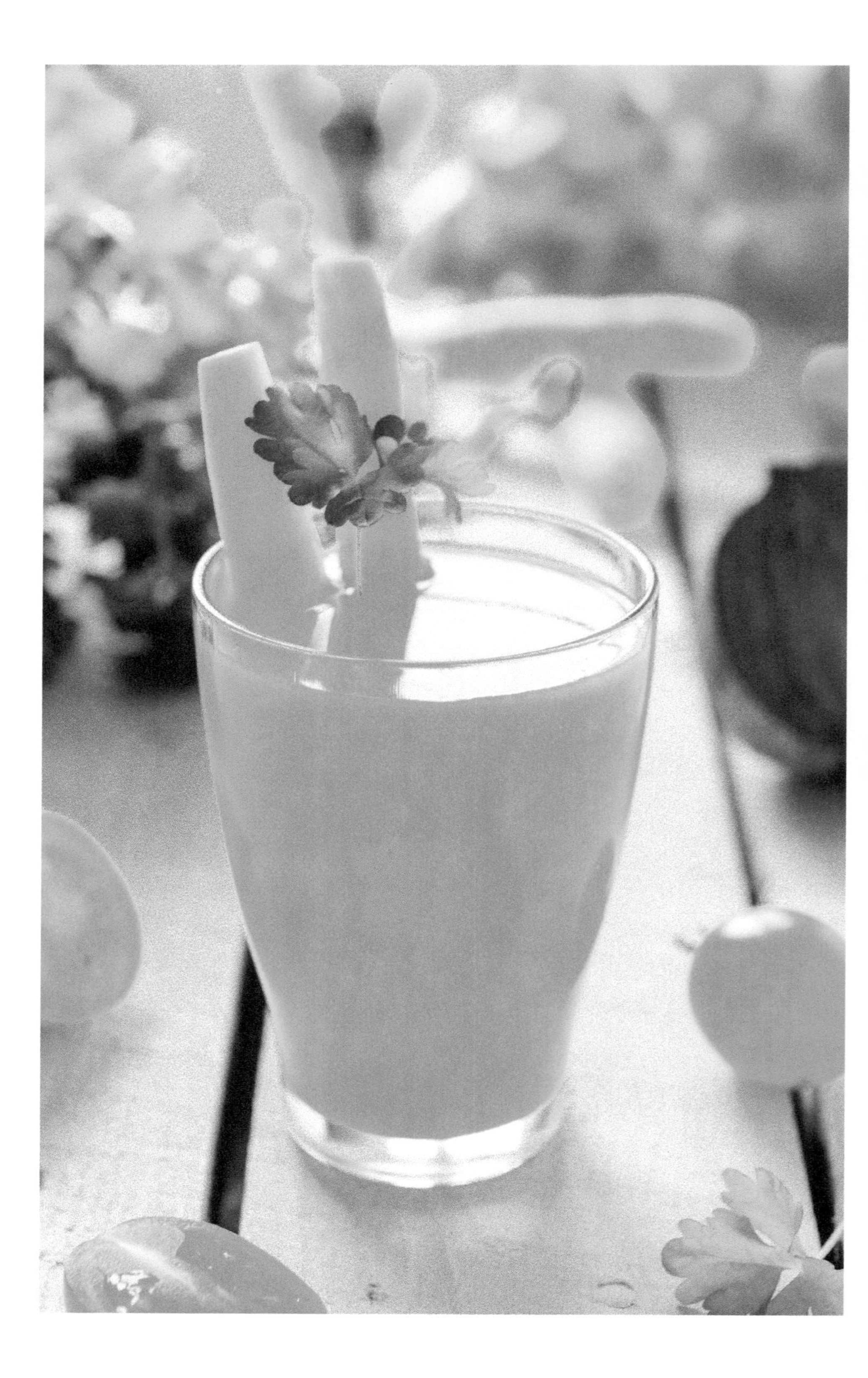

Red Cabbage Carrot Juice

SERVES 2

Cabbage is one of very few vegetables that contain vitamin E. It's also a good source of sulfur, which helps to purify the blood and detoxify the liver.

4 LARGE SWISS CHARD LEAVES
2 LARGE CARROTS
1 MEDIUM APPLE
¼ SMALL HEAD RED CABBAGE
2 TABLESPOONS FRESHLY SQUEEZED LEMON JUICE

1. Peel, cut, deseed, and/or chop the ingredients as needed.
2. Place a container under the juicer's spout.
3. Feed the Swiss chard, carrots, apple, and cabbage through the juicer.
4. Stir the lemon juice into the juice and pour into glasses to serve.

Ginger Green Juice Blend

SERVES 2

Flavored with ginger and sweetened with apple, this juice is something entirely unique and completely refreshing.

1 CUP BABY SPINACH LEAVES
1 LARGE CARROT
1 LARGE STALK CELERY
½ BUNCH KALE LEAVES
½ SMALL CUCUMBER
1 MEDIUM APPLE
1-INCH PIECE GINGERROOT

1. Peel, cut, deseed, and/or chop the ingredients as needed.
2. Place a container under the juicer's spout.
3. Feed the ingredients one at a time, in the order listed, through the juicer.
4. Stir the juice and pour into glasses to serve.

Parsley Power Gulp

SERVES 2

Often used as a garnish rather than an essential ingredient in recipes, parsley actually has a number of significant health benefits. It's an excellent source of folate, which helps to prevent certain cancers, and it has diuretic properties to flush excess water from the body. Parsley is also one of the best natural sources for vitamin C.

1 BUNCH PARSLEY LEAVES
2 MEDIUM CARROTS
2 LARGE STALKS CELERY
1 SMALL APPLE

1. Peel, cut, deseed, and/or chop the ingredients as needed.
2. Place a container under the juicer's spout.
3. Feed the ingredients one at a time, in the order listed, through the juicer.
4. Stir the juice and pour into glasses to serve.

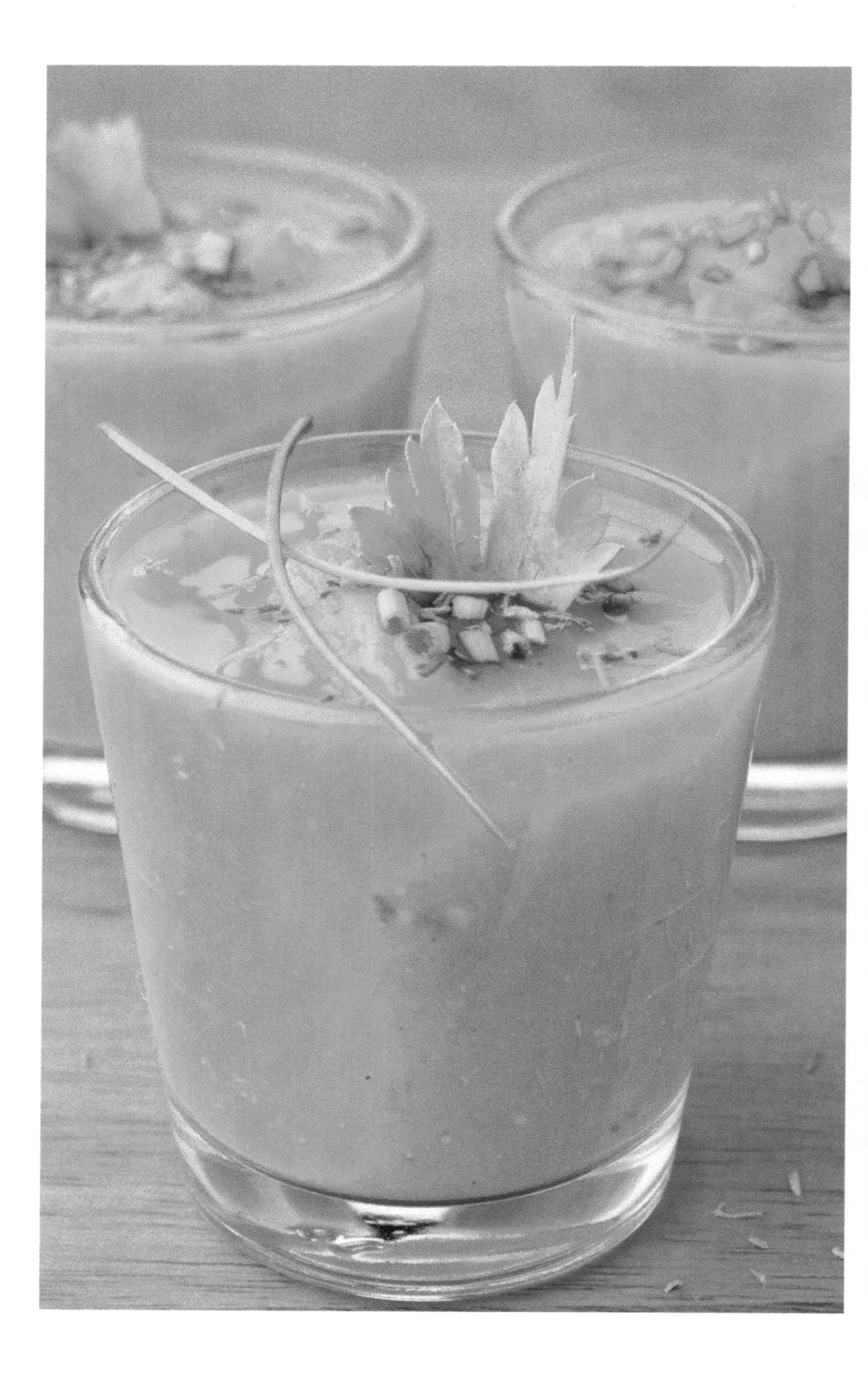

Tomato Gazpacho Juice

SERVES 2

Though gazpacho is traditionally served as a cold soup, in this recipe it transforms into a tasty beverage. Tomatoes contain over nine thousand different phytonutrients, including vitamin C, copper, iron, potassium, and magnesium. They are also a good source of lycopene, which may help prevent cancer and improve mental health.

4 PLUM TOMATOES
2 LARGE STALKS CELERY
1 SEEDLESS CUCUMBER
1 MEDIUM CARROT
1 SMALL RED BELL PEPPER
½ BUNCH PARSLEY LEAVES
1 LIME
1 GREEN ONION

1. Peel, cut, deseed, and/or chop the ingredients as needed.
2. Place a container under the juicer's spout.
3. Feed the ingredients one at a time, in the order listed, through the juicer.
4. Stir the juice and pour into glasses to serve.

Spirulina Avocado Juice

SERVES 2

Though not your typical juice, this spirulina avocado blend is packed with essential nutrients. Avocados are an excellent source of heart-healthy fats as well as potassium, which helps regulate blood pressure. Spirulina, cultivated from algae, helps to boost thyroid function.

2 SMALL APPLES
1 SEEDLESS CUCUMBER
1 RIPE AVOCADO
1 TEASPOON SPIRULINA POWDER

1. Peel, cut, deseed, and/or chop the ingredients as needed.
2. Place a container under the juicer's spout.
3. Feed the apples and cucumber through the juicer.
4. In a blender or food processor, blend the avocado until smooth.
5. Stir the pureed avocado and spirulina into the juice and pour into glasses to serve.

Refreshing Red Bell Pepper Carrot Juice

SERVES 2

Bell peppers are rich in vitamin C, which plays a significant role in eye and gum health. They also contain vitamin A, which is instrumental for healthy skin.

5 MEDIUM CARROTS
3 MEDIUM GREEN APPLES
1 LARGE RED BELL PEPPER

1. Peel, cut, deseed, and/or chop the ingredients as needed.
2. Place a container under the juicer's spout.
3. Feed the ingredients one at a time, in the order listed, through the juicer.
4. Stir the juice and pour into glasses to serve.

Spinach Lime Juice

SERVES 2

If you are in the mood for something fresh and simple, this juice may be just what you need. No muss, no fuss—just delicious.

2 BUNCHES SPINACH LEAVES
1 MEDIUM GREEN APPLE
1 LIME

1. Peel, cut, deseed, and/or chop the ingredients as needed.
2. Place a container under the juicer's spout.
3. Feed the ingredients one at a time, in the order listed, through the juicer.
4. Stir the juice and pour into glasses to serve.

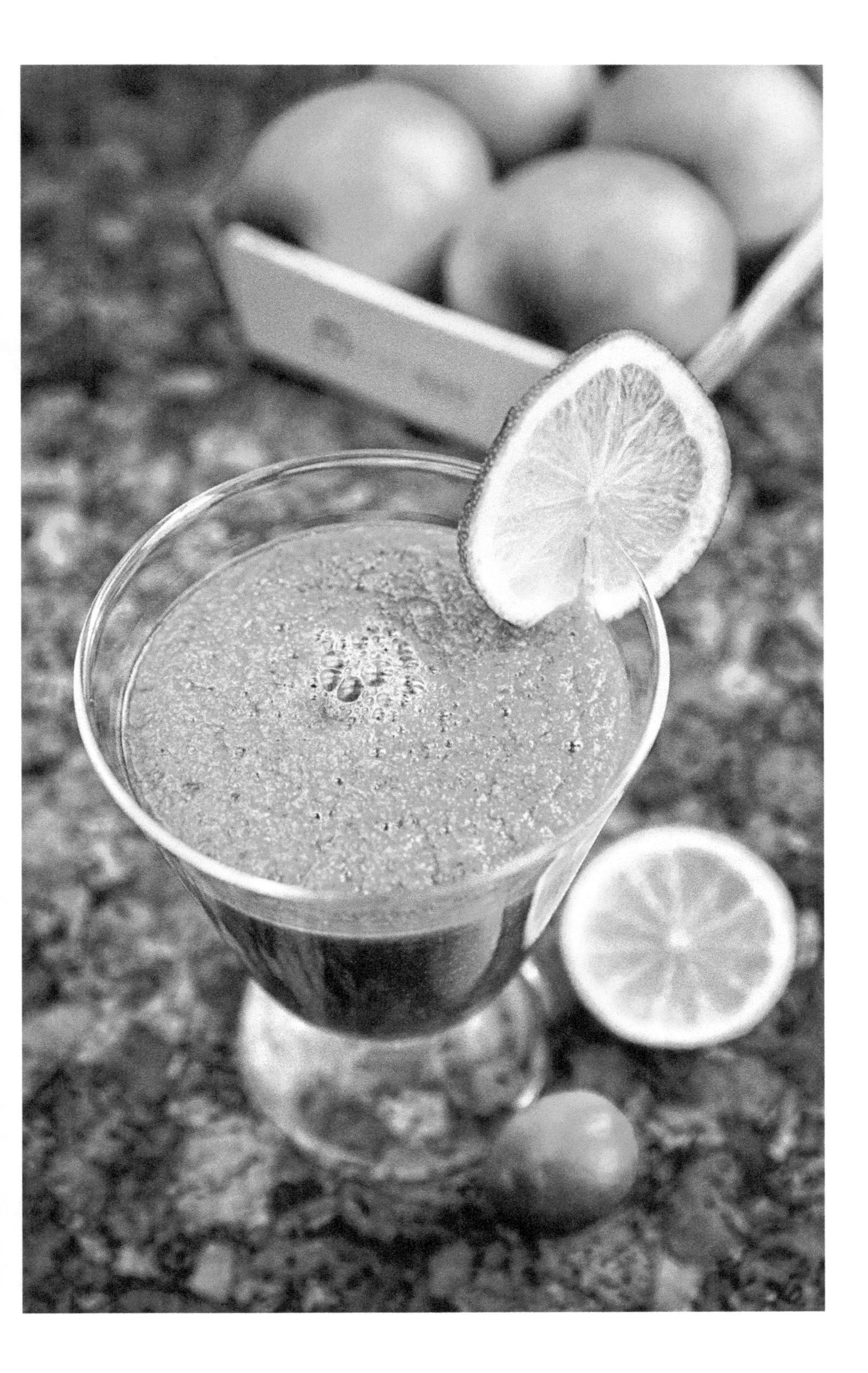

Fabulous Fennel Juice Blend

SERVES 2

Fennel is not a vegetable most people have on their shopping list. Though somewhat uncommon, fennel is an excellent source of nutrition. Loaded with calcium, potassium, phosphorus, and vitamin C, it is particularly beneficial for the digestive system.

2 MEDIUM FENNEL BULBS
1 SMALL STALK CELERY
1 SMALL CARROT
1 MEDIUM APPLE

1. Peel, cut, deseed, and/or chop the ingredients as needed.
2. Place a container under the juicer's spout.
3. Feed the ingredients one at a time, in the order listed, through the juicer.
4. Stir the juice and pour into glasses to serve.

Kick-Start Veggie Juice

SERVES 2

This juice recipe is full of nutritious vegetables to help you kick-start your day. In addition to the health benefits of these vegetables, you also get the crisp, peppery flavor of celery and the freshness of cilantro.

2 LARGE STALKS CELERY
1 LARGE CARROT
½ ROMAINE LETTUCE HEART
½ MEDIUM CUCUMBER
3 SPRIGS CILANTRO

1. Peel, cut, deseed, and/or chop the ingredients as needed.
2. Place a container under the juicer's spout.
3. Feed the ingredients one at a time, in the order listed, through the juicer.
4. Stir the juice and pour into glasses to serve.

Protein Power Juice

SERVES 2

Add a little protein to your favorite juice blends by stirring in a tablespoon of hempseed. Hempseeds are rich in dietary fiber and essential fatty acids. In fact, hempseeds are a more complete protein source than milk, meat, and eggs.

1 BUNCH KALE LEAVES
1 SMALL HEAD BROCCOLI
1 LARGE STALK CELERY
½ BUNCH COLLARD GREENS
1 TABLESPOON HEMPSEED

1. Peel, cut, deseed, and/or chop the ingredients as needed.
2. Place a container under the juicer's spout.
3. Feed the first four ingredients one at a time, in the order listed, through the juicer.
4. Stir the hempseed into the juice and pour into glasses to serve.

Skinny Green Juice

SERVES 2

This skinny juice packs a powerful punch. Made with nutritious, low-calorie ingredients like celery and cucumber, this juice will provide your body with a variety of nutrients without exceeding your calorie goal.

2 LARGE STALKS CELERY
1 CUP ROMAINE LETTUCE
1 CUP BABY SPINACH LEAVES
1 CUP KALE LEAVES
1 SMALL CUCUMBER
6 SPRIGS PARSLEY, DILL, OR CILANTRO
2 TABLESPOONS FRESHLY SQUEEZED LIME JUICE

1. Peel, cut, deseed, and/or chop the ingredients as needed.
2. Place a container under the juicer's spout.
3. Feed the celery, romaine, spinach, kale, cucumber, and parsley, dill, or cilantro through the juicer.
4. Stir the lime juice into the juice and pour into glasses to serve.

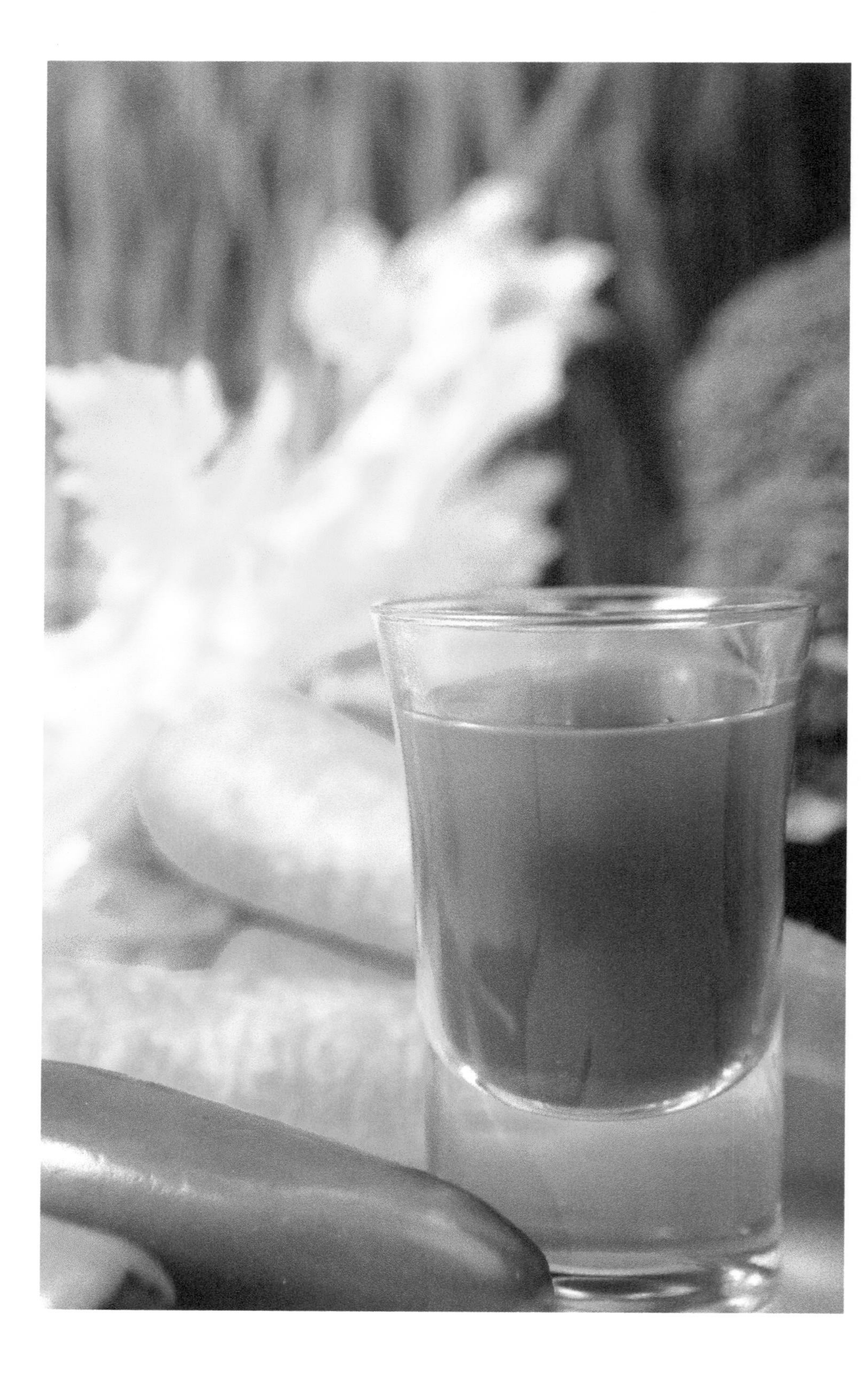

Carrot Celery Cleanse

SERVES 2

Though carrots and celery are the stars of this recipe, the garlic is not to be forgotten. Garlic helps to regulate blood sugar and cholesterol levels while also providing antimicrobial, antibiotic, and anti-cancer properties.

4 LARGE CARROTS
3 LARGE STALKS CELERY
2 LARGE KALE LEAVES
½ BUNCH SPINACH LEAVES
1 CLOVE GARLIC
1 GREEN CHILI

1. Peel, cut, deseed, and/or chop the ingredients as needed.
2. Place a container under the juicer's spout.
3. Feed the ingredients one at a time, in the order listed, through the juicer.
4. Stir the juice and pour into glasses to serve.

Breakfast of Champions Juice

SERVES 2

Carrots are not only the most readily available vegetable, they are also incredibly rich in vitamins and minerals. In addition, carrots also contain beta-carotene and carotenoids, which help reduce the risk for cancer and cardiovascular disease.

6 MEDIUM CARROTS
2 SMALL BEETS
2 MEDIUM APPLES
2 CUPS PACKED BABY SPINACH LEAVES
¼ CUP MINT LEAVES

1. Peel, cut, deseed, and/or chop the ingredients as needed.
2. Place a container under the juicer's spout.
3. Feed the ingredients one at a time, in the order listed, through the juicer.
4. Stir the juice and pour into glasses to serve.

Green Garden Delight

SERVES 2

This recipe is loaded with healthy vegetables, including carrots, celery, bell pepper, and spinach. Spinach is known for its choline content. Choline is a B-complex vitamin that supports cognitive function. These benefits, combined with the nutrients in the other ingredients, create a juice that is perfectly delightful.

2 CUPS BABY SPINACH LEAVES
1 LARGE CARROT
1 LARGE STALK CELERY
½ MEDIUM GREEN BELL PEPPER
½ BUNCH PARSLEY
½ BUNCH CILANTRO

1. Peel, cut, deseed, and/or chop the ingredients as needed.
2. Place a container under the juicer's spout.
3. Feed the ingredients one at a time, in the order listed, through the juicer.
4. Stir the juice and pour into glasses to serve.

Pumpkin Pie Juice

SERVES 2

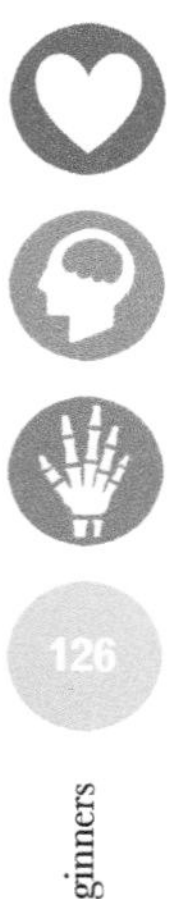

Rather than reaching for that extra slice of pumpkin pie, try this juice instead! Pumpkin is an excellent source of vitamins C and E, and it also has anti-inflammatory and blood-sugar stabilizing properties.

2 CUPS PUMPKIN
2 MEDIUM APPLES
1 CUP COLD WATER
1 TEASPOON PUMPKIN PIE SPICE
1 TEASPOON RAW HONEY

1. Peel, cut, deseed, and/or chop the ingredients as needed.
2. Place a container under the juicer's spout.
3. Feed the pumpkin and apples through the juicer.
4. Stir the water, pumpkin pie spice, and honey into the juice and pour into glasses to serve.

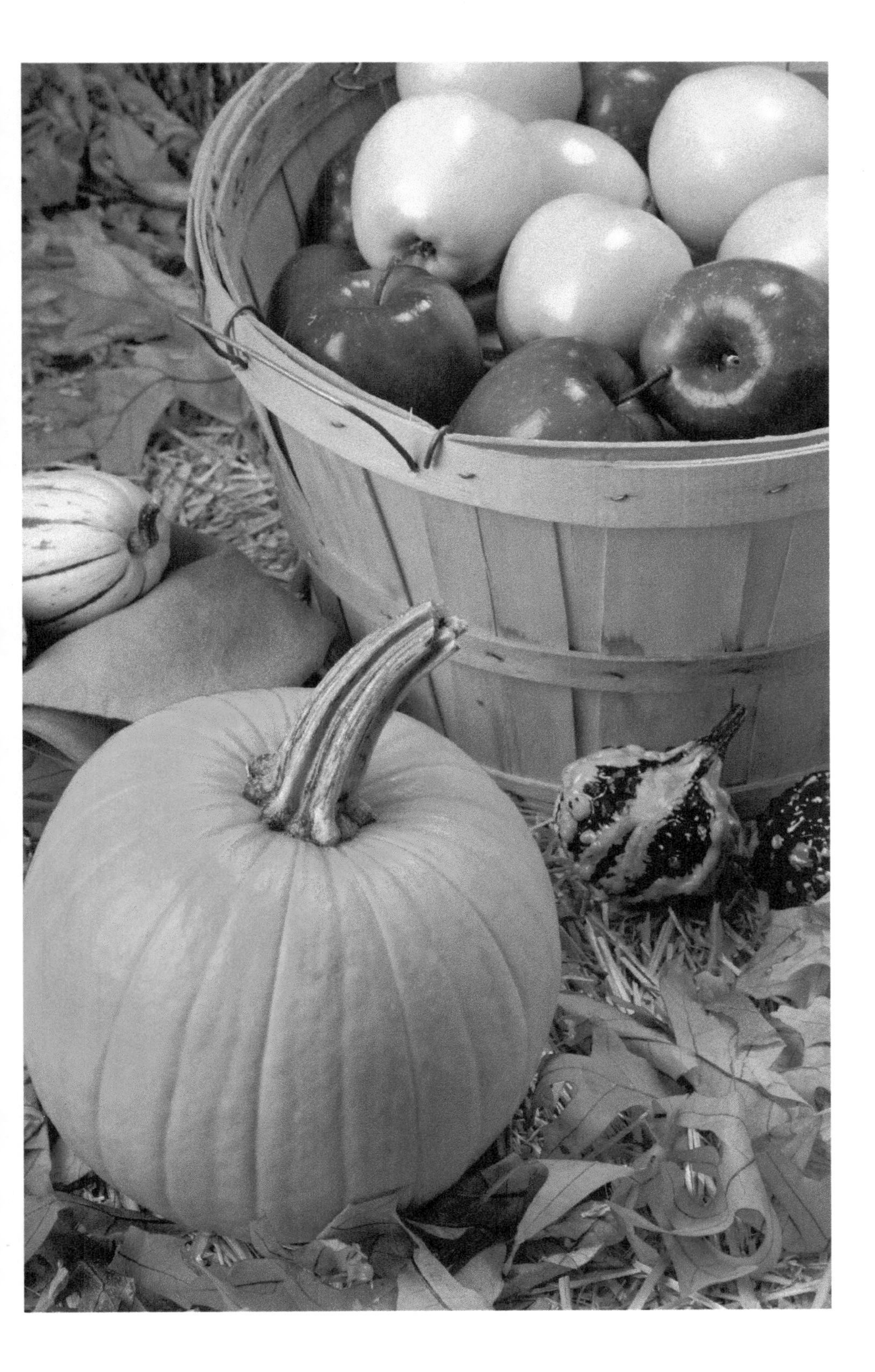

Liver Detox Tonic

SERVES 2

Ginger is highly valued for its detoxification properties. In this recipe, it marries perfectly with the nutrients found in kale and bok choy to create a delicious drink that's almost too good to be true.

1 SMALL BABY BOK CHOY
3 LARGE KALE LEAVES
1 MEDIUM APPLE
1 SMALL LEMON
½-INCH PIECE GINGERROOT

1. Peel, cut, deseed, and/or chop the ingredients as needed.
2. Place a container under the juicer's spout.
3. Feed the ingredients one at a time, in the order listed, through the juicer.
4. Stir the juice and pour into glasses to serve.

Cucumber Wake-Up Call

SERVES 2

Cucumbers are a good source of B vitamins, which help to regulate blood pressure. Combined with hearty kale, spinach, and the light sweetness of apple, this juice will give you something to wake up for.

2 MEDIUM CUCUMBERS
2 LARGE KALE LEAVES
1 CUP BABY SPINACH LEAVES
1 MEDIUM APPLE

1. Peel, cut, deseed, and/or chop the ingredients as needed.
2. Place a container under the juicer's spout.
3. Feed the ingredients one at a time, in the order listed, through the juicer.
4. Stir the juice and pour into glasses to serve.

Best Foot Forward Juice

SERVES 2

Parsnips are valued for their anti-cancer properties as well as their high levels of iron and calcium. Together with carrots, celery, and cucumber, they help this juice provide you with the nutrition needed to get your day off to a wonderful start.

2 LARGE CARROTS
1 LARGE STALK CELERY
1 MEDIUM CUCUMBER
1 PARSNIP WITH GREENS
½ LEMON

1. Peel, cut, deseed, and/or chop the ingredients as needed.
2. Place a container under the juicer's spout.
3. Feed the ingredients one at a time, in the order listed, through the juicer.
4. Stir the juice and pour into glasses to serve.

Minty Mojito Juice

SERVES 2

The fresh herbs in this juice combine beautifully with zesty lime. If you are craving that mojito flavor, but would rather go for something a little more nutritious, try this!

1 MEDIUM CUCUMBER
½ CUP PACKED MINT LEAVES
½ CUP PACKED BASIL LEAVES
1 MEDIUM APPLE
1 LIME

1. Peel, cut, deseed, and/or chop the ingredients as needed.
2. Place a container under the juicer's spout.
3. Feed the ingredients one at a time, in the order listed, through the juicer.
4. Stir the juice and pour into glasses to serve.

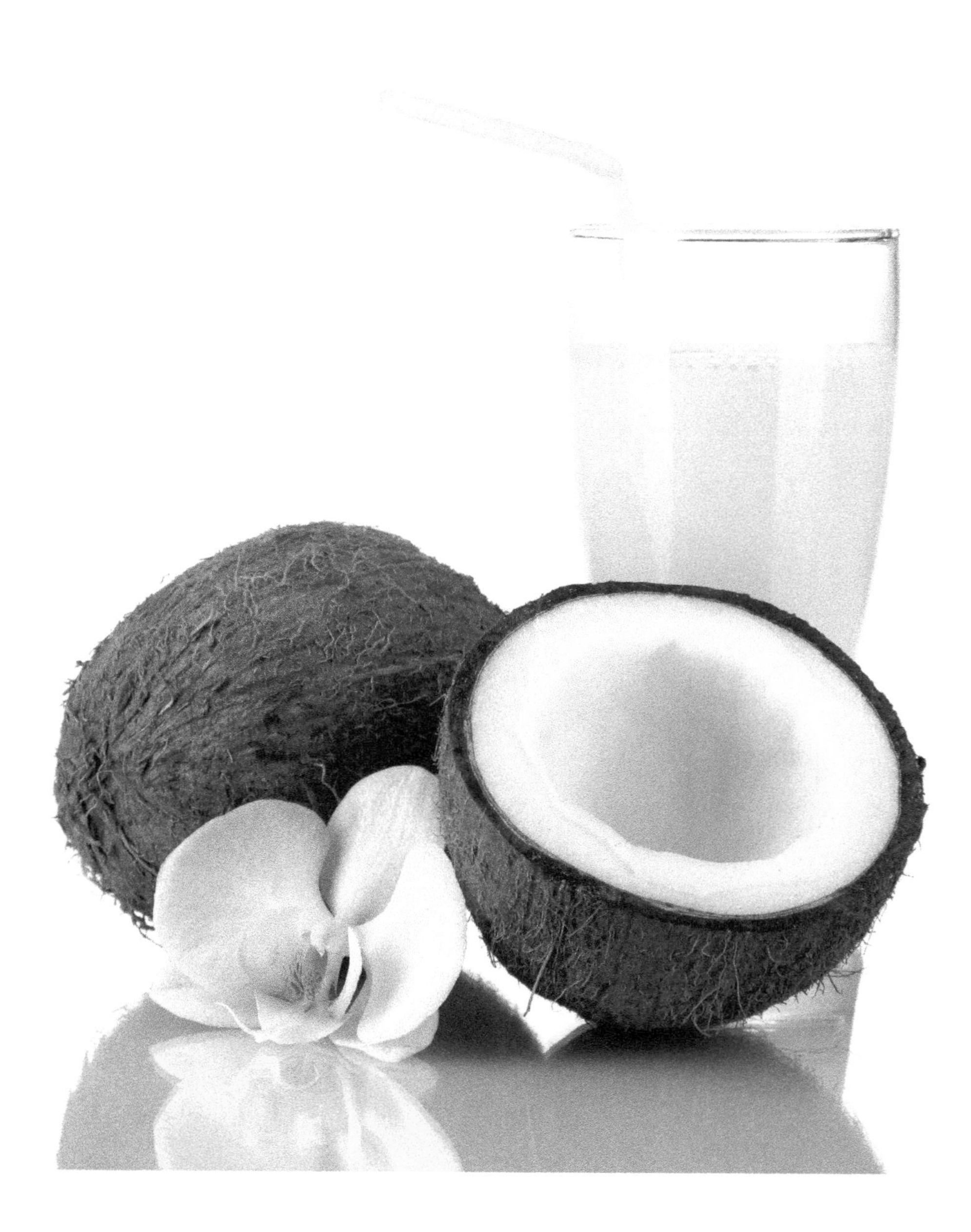

Cool Cilantro Coconut Juice

SERVES 3

This cool juice is just what you need on a hot summer day. Enjoy it while relaxing by the pool, or use it to rehydrate your body after a tough workout.

½ BUNCH CILANTRO
½ LIME
4 CUPS COCONUT WATER

1. Peel, cut, deseed, and/or chop the ingredients as needed.
2. Place a container under the juicer's spout.
3. Feed the cilantro and lime through the juicer.
4. Stir the coconut water into the juice and pour into glasses to serve.

Summer Squash Supreme

SERVES 2

Summer squash is not a vegetable you often see in juicing recipes. It makes a wonderful addition, however, because it is low in calories but high in antioxidants that help repair damage caused by free radicals.

4 CUPS SUMMER SQUASH
1 LARGE APPLE
2 CINNAMON STICKS

1. Peel, cut, deseed, and/or chop the ingredients as needed.
2. Place a container under the juicer's spout.
3. Feed the squash and apple through the juicer.
4. Pour into glasses and serve with the cinnamon sticks.

Beet Berry Blast

SERVES 2

This juice recipe is the perfect combination of nutritious vegetables and fresh fruit flavor. Topped off with a handful of cilantro, this juice is both healthy and refreshing!

3 MEDIUM BEETS
2 LARGE STALKS CELERY
1½ CUPS MIXED BERRIES
1 MEDIUM APPLE
½ BUNCH CILANTRO LEAVES

1. Peel, cut, deseed, and/or chop the ingredients as needed.
2. Place a container under the juicer's spout.
3. Feed the ingredients one at a time, in the order listed, through the juicer.
4. Stir the juice and pour into glasses to serve.

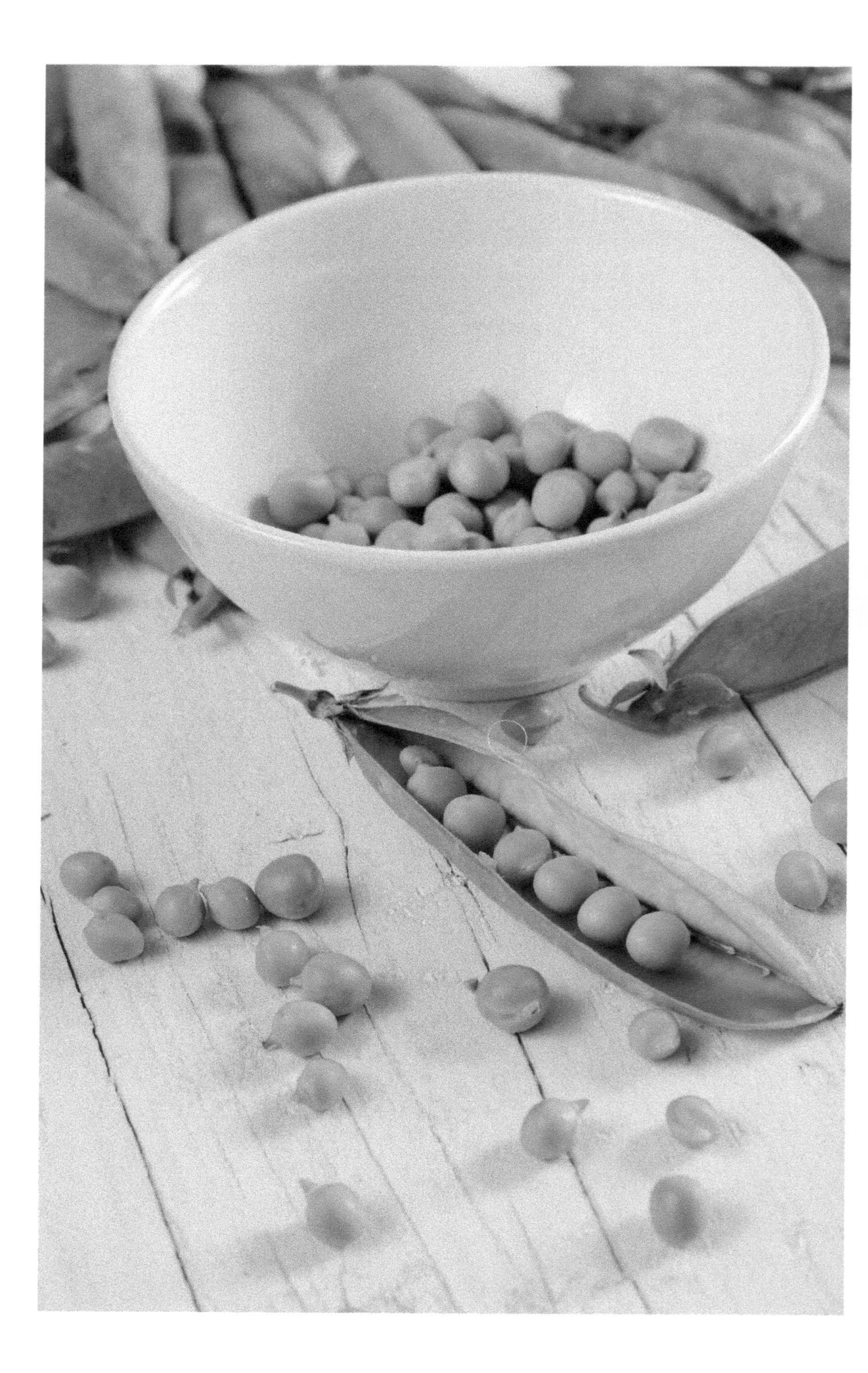

CHAPTER NINE

Green Juices

"There's a major distinction between pasteurized juice and cold-pressed juice. . . . When juice is pasteurized, it's heated at a very high temperature, which protects it against bacteria and prolongs shelf life. However, this heating process also destroys live enzymes, minerals, and other beneficial nutrients. Cold pressing . . . extracts juice by crushing the fruits and vegetables . . . all without using heat."

—KERI GLASSMAN, R.D.

Health-Benefit Icons

Each juice recipe includes the top 3 benefits based on the nutritional and health information presented in Chapters 2, 3, and 4. Use the following icons as a guide.

HEALTHY DIGESTION

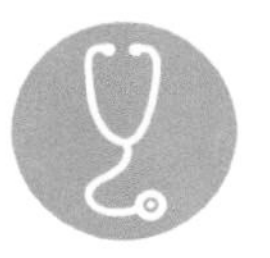
ANTI-CANCER

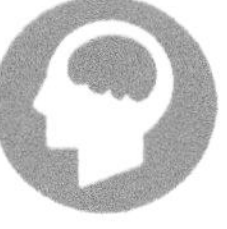
BRAIN HEALTH

HEART HEALTH

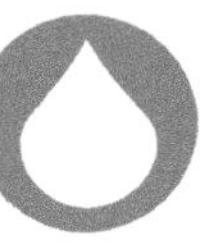
CLEANSE & DETOX

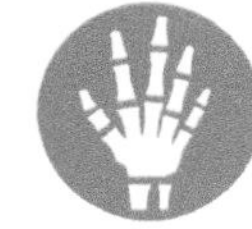
BONE & BLOOD HEALTH

Green Goodness Juice

SERVES 2

This juice is aptly named because it is, after all, full of green goodness. With ingredients like cabbage, cucumber, kale, and green bell pepper, this juice is nothing short of amazing.

1 CUP CARROTS
1 CUP GREEN, RED, OR SAVOY CABBAGE
1 SMALL CUCUMBER
1 SMALL GREEN BELL PEPPER
1 LARGE KALE LEAF
1 SMALL BUNCH CILANTRO

1. Peel, cut, deseed, and/or chop the ingredients as needed.
2. Place a container under the juicer's spout.
3. Feed the ingredients one at a time, in the order listed, through the juicer.
4. Stir the juice and pour into glasses to serve.

Glorious Green Juice

SERVES 2

As a low-calorie ingredient, celery is excellent in any green juice. Celery is also a good source of silicon, which helps strengthen bones and joints.

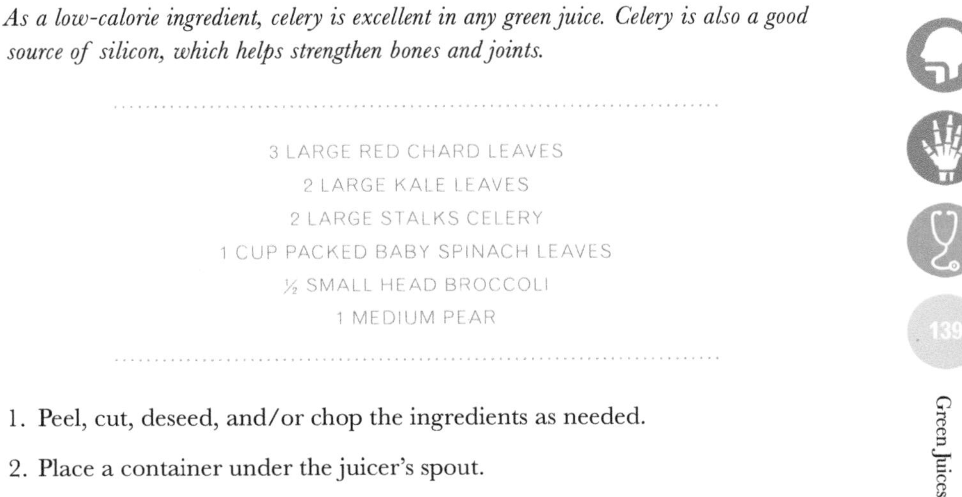

3 LARGE RED CHARD LEAVES
2 LARGE KALE LEAVES
2 LARGE STALKS CELERY
1 CUP PACKED BABY SPINACH LEAVES
½ SMALL HEAD BROCCOLI
1 MEDIUM PEAR

1. Peel, cut, deseed, and/or chop the ingredients as needed.
2. Place a container under the juicer's spout.
3. Feed the ingredients one at a time, in the order listed, through the juicer.
4. Stir the juice and pour into glasses to serve.

Beautiful Beet Juice

SERVES 2

When you hear the word "beauty," beets may not be what come, to mind. Beet greens are, however, loaded with healthy vitamins and minerals that will rejuvenate your body and your appearance.

2 CUPS BEET GREENS
½ SMALL CUCUMBER
½ SMALL HEAD GREEN CABBAGE
½ BUNCH PARSLEY

1. Peel, cut, deseed, and/or chop the ingredients as needed.
2. Place a container under the juicer's spout.
3. Feed the ingredients one at a time, in the order listed, through the juicer.
4. Stir the juice and pour into glasses to serve.

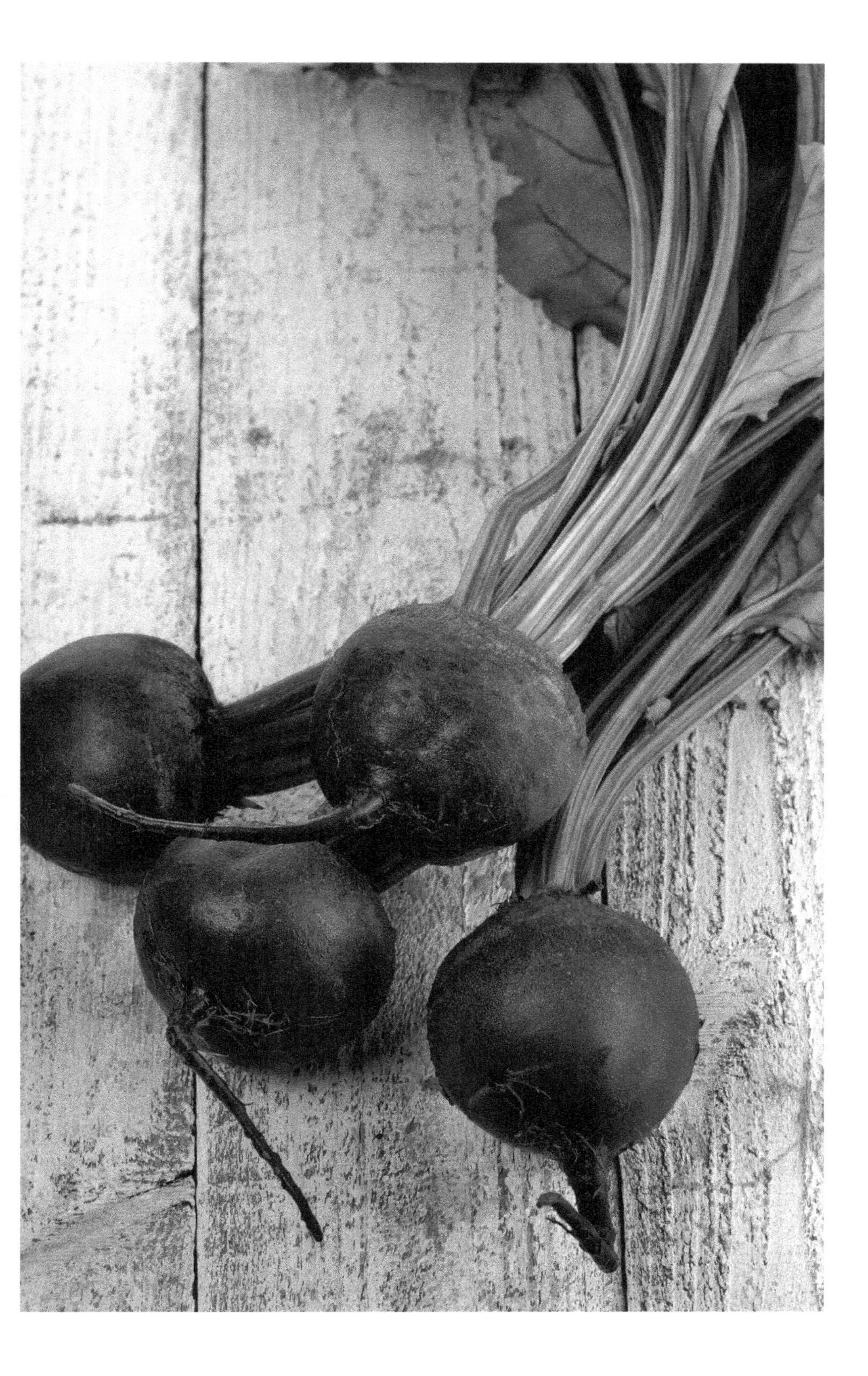

Green Good Morning Juice

SERVES 2

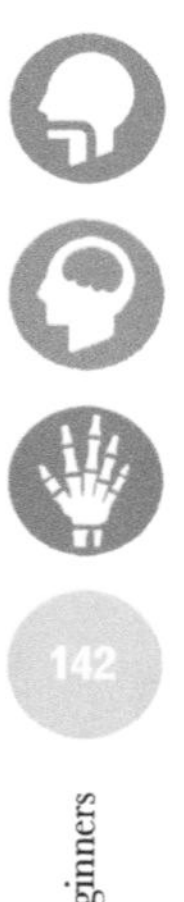

This juice is loaded with leafy greens to help you start your day off right. Romaine lettuce is rich in vitamins C, A, and K, as well as minerals, including iron, potassium, magnesium, and manganese.

½ BUNCH SPINACH LEAVES
2 LARGE ROMAINE LETTUCE LEAVES
2 LARGE SWISS CHARD LEAVES
2 SMALL CUCUMBERS
1 SMALL APPLE
1-INCH PIECE GINGERROOT

1. Peel, cut, deseed, and/or chop the ingredients as needed.
2. Place a container under the juicer's spout.
3. Feed the ingredients one at a time, in the order listed, through the juicer.
4. Stir the juice and pour into glasses to serve.

Seven-Layer Green Juice

SERVES 2

Seven nutritious ingredients, one delicious beverage. The beauty of this green juice is that you can mix and match whatever vegetables you have on hand to create your own flavor combinations!

1 CUP GREEN CABBAGE
1 LARGE STALK CELERY
1 SMALL SWEET POTATO
½ SMALL CUCUMBER
½ SMALL GREEN BELL PEPPER
½ CUP FENNEL BULB
1-INCH PIECE GINGERROOT

1. Peel, cut, deseed, and/or chop the ingredients as needed.
2. Place a container under the juicer's spout.
3. Feed the ingredients one at a time, in the order listed, through the juicer.
4. Stir the juice and pour into glasses to serve.

Dreamy Green Juice

SERVES 3

Packed with all the nutritious goodness of kale, zucchini, and broccoli, this juice is positively dreamy.

4 LARGE CURLY KALE LEAVES
3 MEDIUM APPLES
1 MEDIUM ZUCCHINI
1 SMALL HEAD BROCCOLI

1. Peel, cut, deseed, and/or chop the ingredients as needed.
2. Place a container under the juicer's spout.
3. Feed the ingredients one at a time, in the order listed, through the juicer.
4. Stir the juice and pour into glasses to serve.

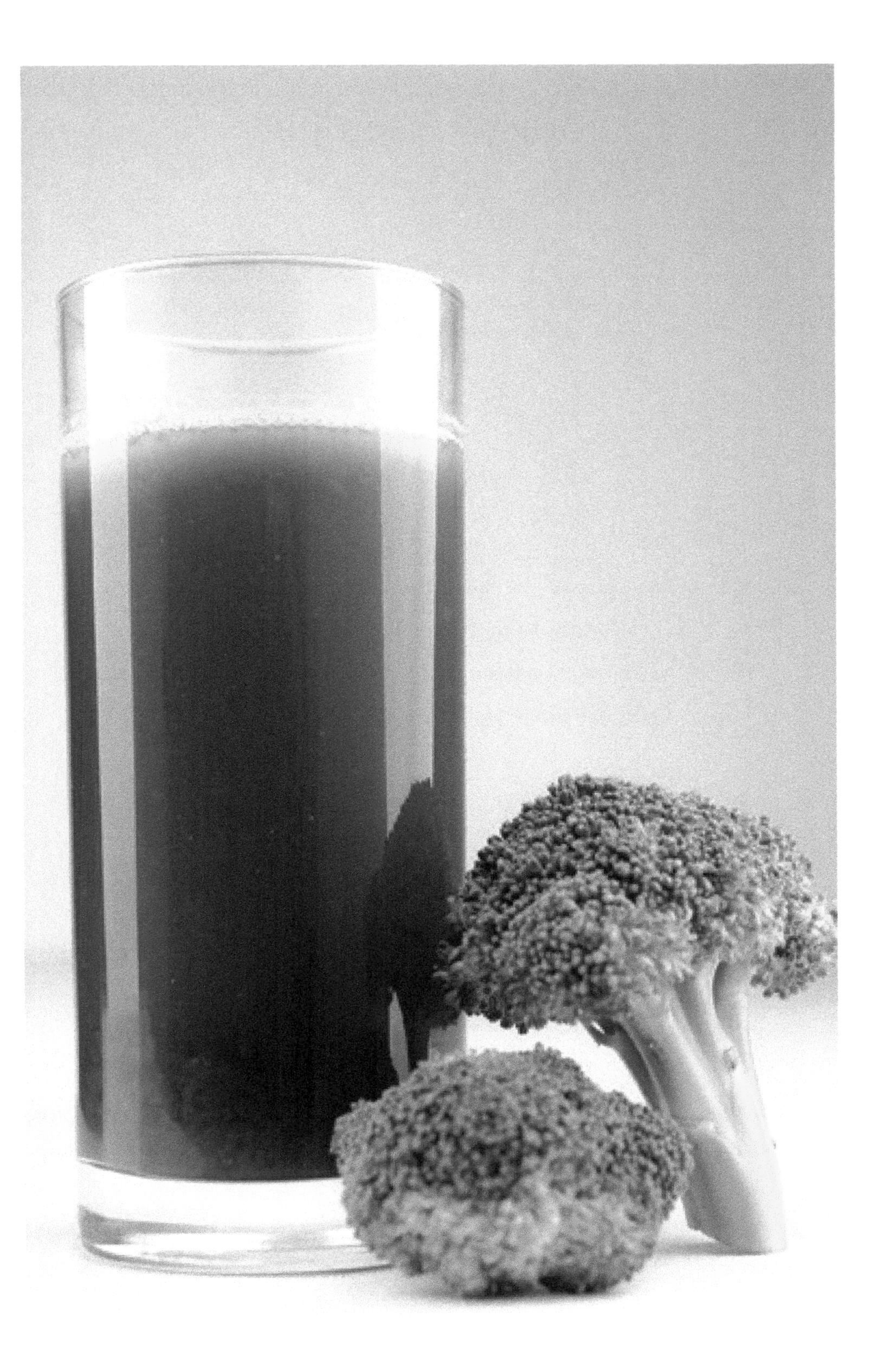

Spicy Green Juice

SERVES 2

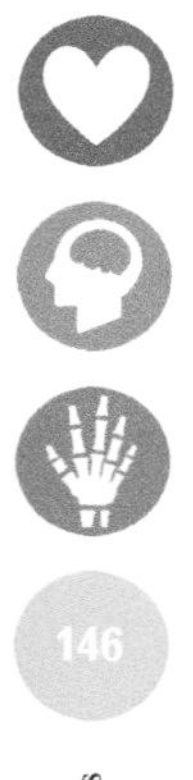

If you are looking for a juice that has a little kick, then look no further. In addition to its spicy flavor, ginger is also known for its detoxification benefits. This root has anti-inflammatory properties and it will help to support healthy digestion.

4 LARGE SWISS CHARD LEAVES
4 LARGE COLLARD GREEN LEAVES
1 SMALL HEAD GREEN CABBAGE
1-INCH PIECE GINGERROOT

1. Peel, cut, deseed, and/or chop the ingredients as needed.
2. Place a container under the juicer's spout.
3. Feed the ingredients one at a time, in the order listed, through the juicer.
4. Stir the juice and pour into glasses to serve.

Mango Tango Green Juice

SERVES 2

If eating vegetables is a chore, this juice will let you off the hook. You still get the nutritional benefits of vegetables like kale and spinach, but all you taste is the sweet flavor of mango.

4 LARGE KALE LEAVES
3 LARGE STALKS CELERY
1 RIPE MANGO
1 SMALL BUNCH SPINACH LEAVES

1. Peel, cut, deseed, and/or chop the ingredients as needed.
2. Place a container under the juicer's spout.
3. Feed the ingredients one at a time, in the order listed, through the juicer.
4. Stir the juice and pour into glasses to serve.

Brilliant Brussels Juice

SERVES 2

Brussels sprouts have been linked to cancer prevention and they are also known to support body detoxification. These vegetables are also rich in vitamins and minerals. In fact, a single cup of Brussels sprouts contains your entire daily value of vitamins C and K.

12 BRUSSELS SPROUTS
4 LARGE KALE LEAVES
1 LARGE APPLE

1. Peel, cut, deseed, and/or chop the ingredients as needed.
2. Place a container under the juicer's spout.
3. Feed the ingredients one at a time, in the order listed, through the juicer.
4. Stir the juice and pour into glasses to serve.

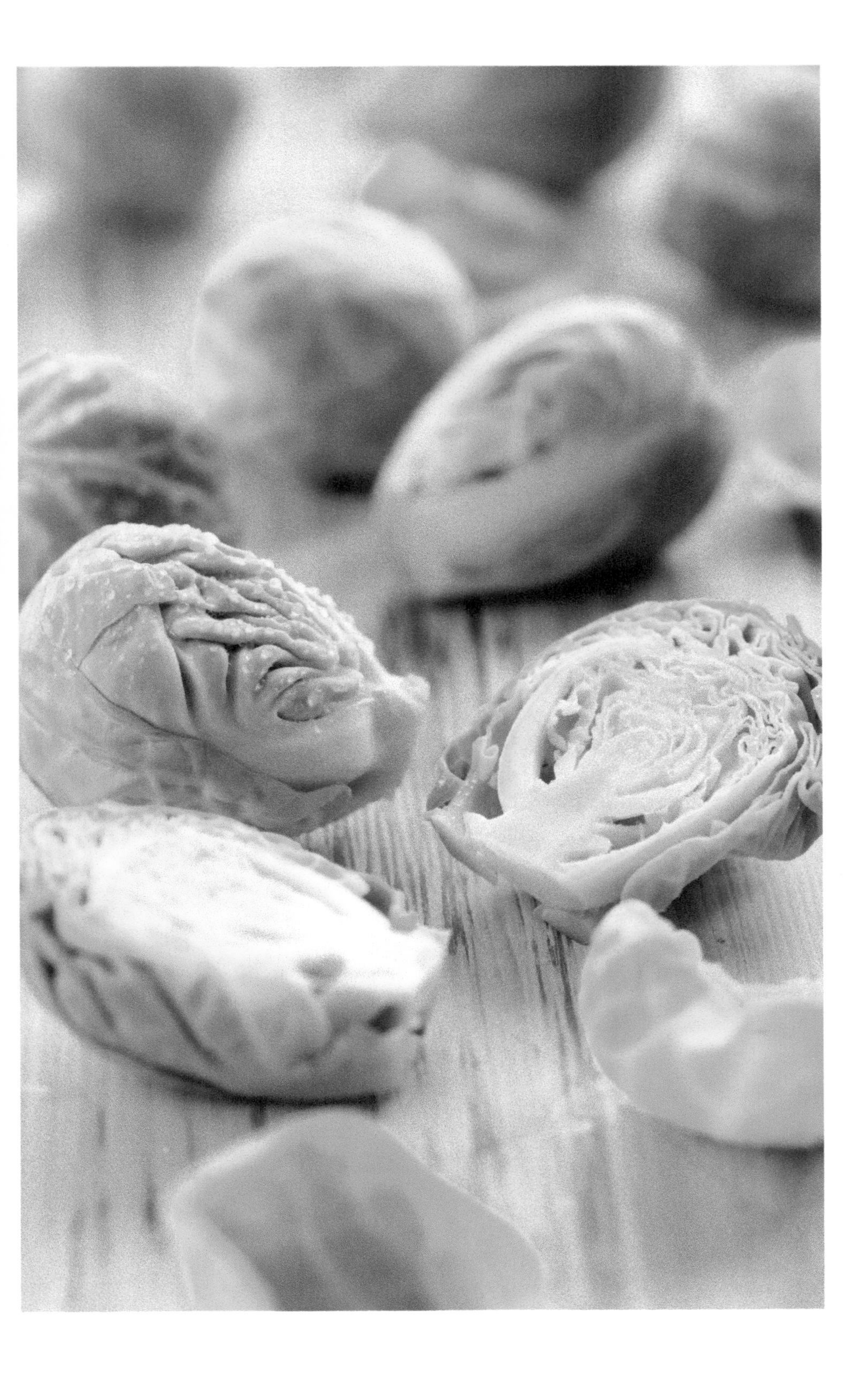

Easy Peasy Green Lemonade

SERVES 2

This scrumptious green juice combines the refreshing taste of lemonade with the many health benefits of melon, asparagus, and pear.

1 SMALL HONEYDEW MELON
1 BUNCH ASPARAGUS
1 MEDIUM PEAR
1 LEMON

1. Peel, cut, deseed, and/or chop the ingredients as needed.
2. Place a container under the juicer's spout.
3. Feed the ingredients one at a time, in the order listed, through the juicer.
4. Stir the juice and pour into glasses to serve.

Double Trouble Broccoli Juice

SERVES 2

Broccoli rabe is a cruciferous vegetable that resembles broccoli but doesn't form a large head. The leaves, buds, and stems are edible, and along with broccoli, all contain high levels of dietary fiber, iron, potassium, and vitamins C and E.

1 SMALL HEAD BROCCOLI
1 BUNCH BROCCOLI RABE
1 LARGE APPLE
1 CLOVE GARLIC

1. Peel, cut, deseed, and/or chop the ingredients as needed.
2. Place a container under the juicer's spout.
3. Feed the ingredients one at a time, in the order listed, through the juicer.
4. Stir the juice and pour into glasses to serve.

Merry Melon Dream Juice

SERVES 2

Fennel is known for its beneficial effects on the digestive system as well as its vitamin and mineral content. In this recipe, the rich flavors of fennel and asparagus are perfectly complemented by the light sweetness of cantaloupe.

4 LARGE KALE LEAVES
½ BUNCH ASPARAGUS
½ RIPE CANTALOUPE
½ FENNEL BULB

1. Peel, cut, deseed, and/or chop the ingredients as needed.
2. Place a container under the juicer's spout.
3. Feed the ingredients one at a time, in the order listed, through the juicer.
4. Stir the juice and pour into glasses to serve.

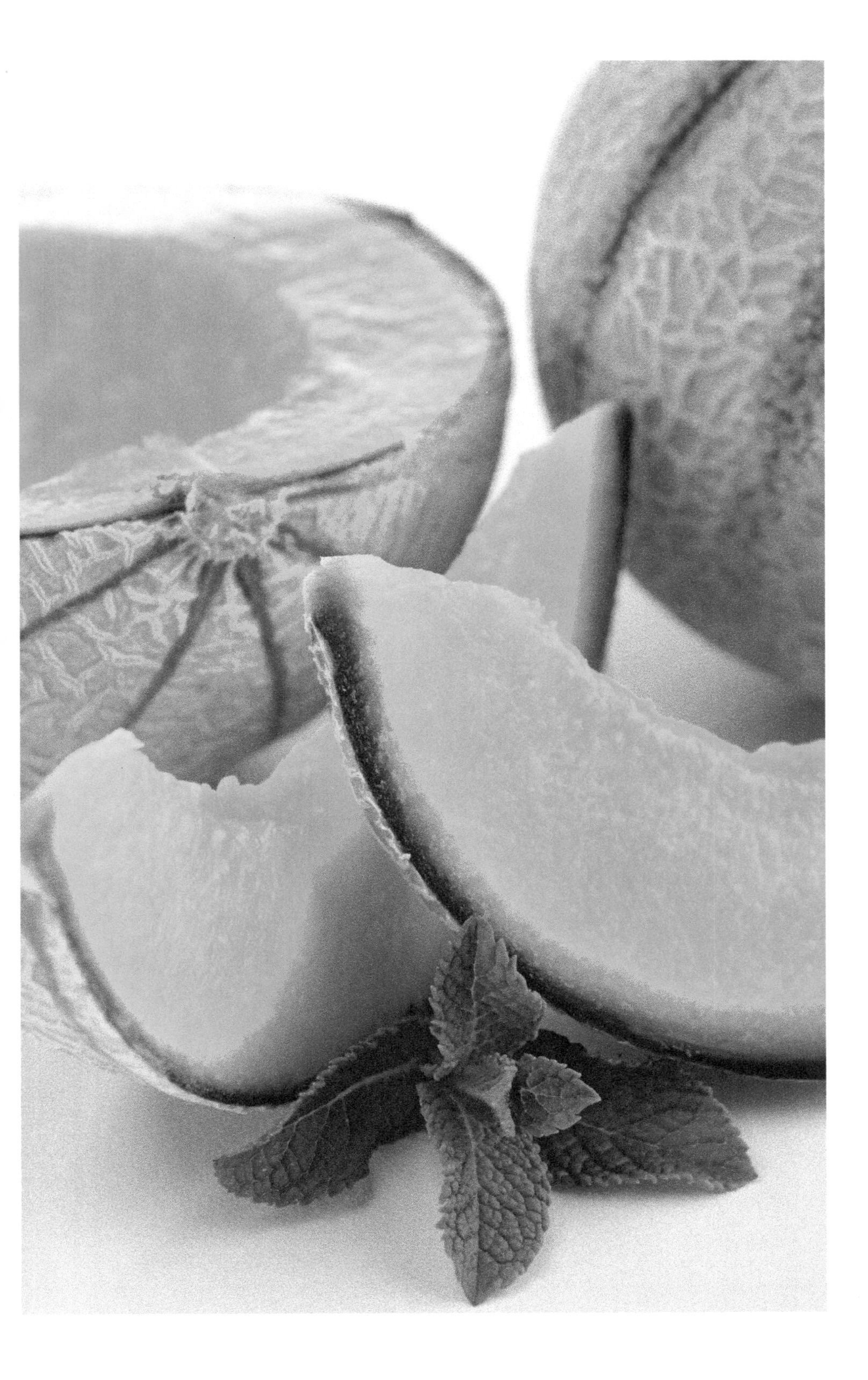

Sensibly Sweet Juice

SERVES 2

If you aren't a fan of overly sweetened juice, this pleasantly mild one may be the right choice for you. With only three ingredients, it is simple and simply delicious.

6 LARGE STALKS CELERY
½ HEAD ROMAINE LETTUCE
1 LARGE APPLE

1. Peel, cut, deseed, and/or chop the ingredients as needed.
2. Place a container under the juicer's spout.
3. Feed the ingredients one at a time, in the order listed, through the juicer.
4. Stir the juice and pour into glasses to serve.

Tossed Salad Juice

SERVES 3

If you don't have time to sit down to eat a salad, this salad-inspired juice is just as good—or even better! With all of the ingredients you would find in a tossed salad, this refreshing beverage will satisfy your hunger and fill your body with healthy nutrients.

1 ROMAINE LETTUCE HEART
6 MEDIUM CARROTS
3 MEDIUM STALKS CELERY
1 MEDIUM CUCUMBER
1 CLOVE GARLIC

1. Peel, cut, deseed, and/or chop the ingredients as needed.
2. Place a container under the juicer's spout.
3. Feed the ingredients one at a time, in the order listed, through the juicer.
4. Stir the juice and pour into glasses to serve.

Cool Cauliflower Juice

SERVES 3

Cauliflower is rich in phosphorus, potassium, manganese, and vitamin K. It is also a good source of glucosinolates, which help support your liver in its natural detoxification abilities.

12 BRUSSELS SPROUTS
1 SMALL HEAD CAULIFLOWER
3 RADISHES WITH GREENS
1 LARGE CARROT
½ SMALL HEAD GREEN CABBAGE

1. Peel, cut, deseed, and/or chop the ingredients as needed.
2. Place a container under the juicer's spout.
3. Feed the ingredients one at a time, in the order listed, through the juicer.
4. Stir the juice and pour into glasses to serve.

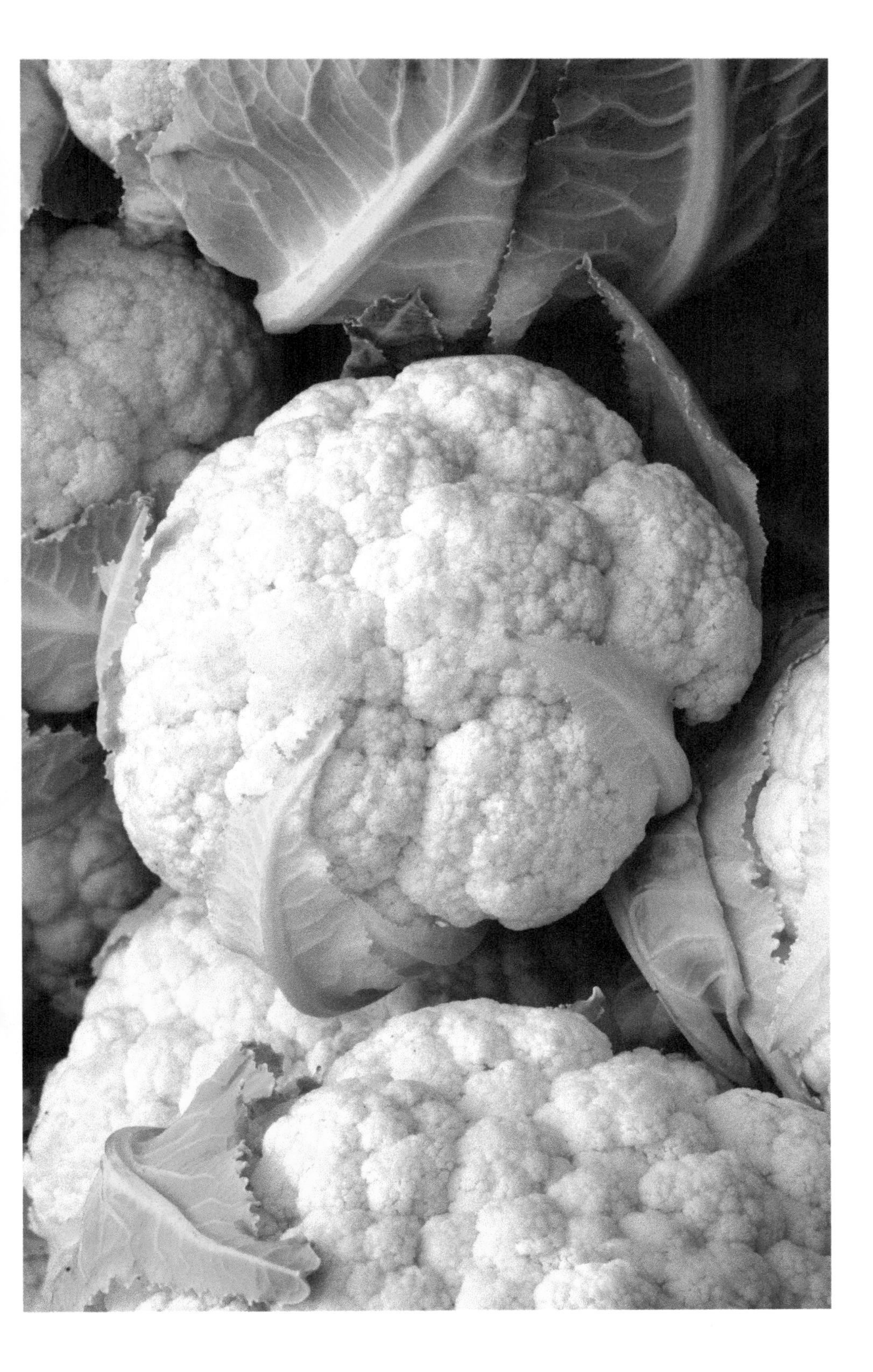

Refreshing Green Juice

SERVES 3

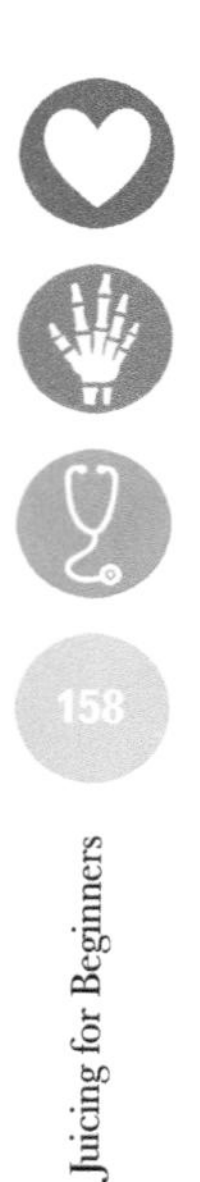

This recipe combines the crispness of bell pepper and cucumber with the fresh bite of cilantro to create an utterly refreshing juice.

6 MEDIUM CARROTS
2 LARGE STALKS CELERY WITH LEAVES
1 BUNCH CILANTRO
1 MEDIUM GREEN BELL PEPPER
1 MEDIUM CUCUMBER
½ BUNCH SPINACH LEAVES
1 CLOVE GARLIC

1. Peel, cut, deseed, and/or chop the ingredients as needed.
2. Place a container under the juicer's spout.
3. Feed the ingredients one at a time, in the order listed, through the juicer.
4. Stir the juice and pour into glasses to serve.

Deeply Green Juice

SERVES 3

This recipe yields a nutritious juice with a beautiful deep green color. Most of this color can be attributed to kale, which has the highest vegetable source of vitamin K.

1 BUNCH CURLY KALE LEAVES
1 BUNCH DANDELION GREENS
3 SPRIGS PARSLEY
1 LARGE APPLE
½ MEDIUM HEAD CABBAGE

1. Peel, cut, deseed, and/or chop the ingredients as needed.
2. Place a container under the juicer's spout.
3. Feed the ingredients one at a time, in the order listed, through the juicer.
4. Stir the juice and pour into glasses to serve.

Rocket Fuel Green Juice

SERVES 3

Blast off with this delectable, nutrient-packed green juice. Made with fresh greens such as arugula and kale, this juice has all the nutrients you need to start your day. Arugula, for example, is loaded with flavonoids, which help reduce cancer risk.

1 BUNCH ARUGULA
½ BUNCH KALE LEAVES
6 MEDIUM CARROTS
2 MEDIUM APPLES
1 RED CHILI PEPPER
1 CLOVE GARLIC

1. Peel, cut, deseed, and/or chop the ingredients as needed.
2. Place a container under the juicer's spout.
3. Feed the ingredients one at a time, in the order listed, through the juicer.
4. Stir the juice and pour into glasses to serve.

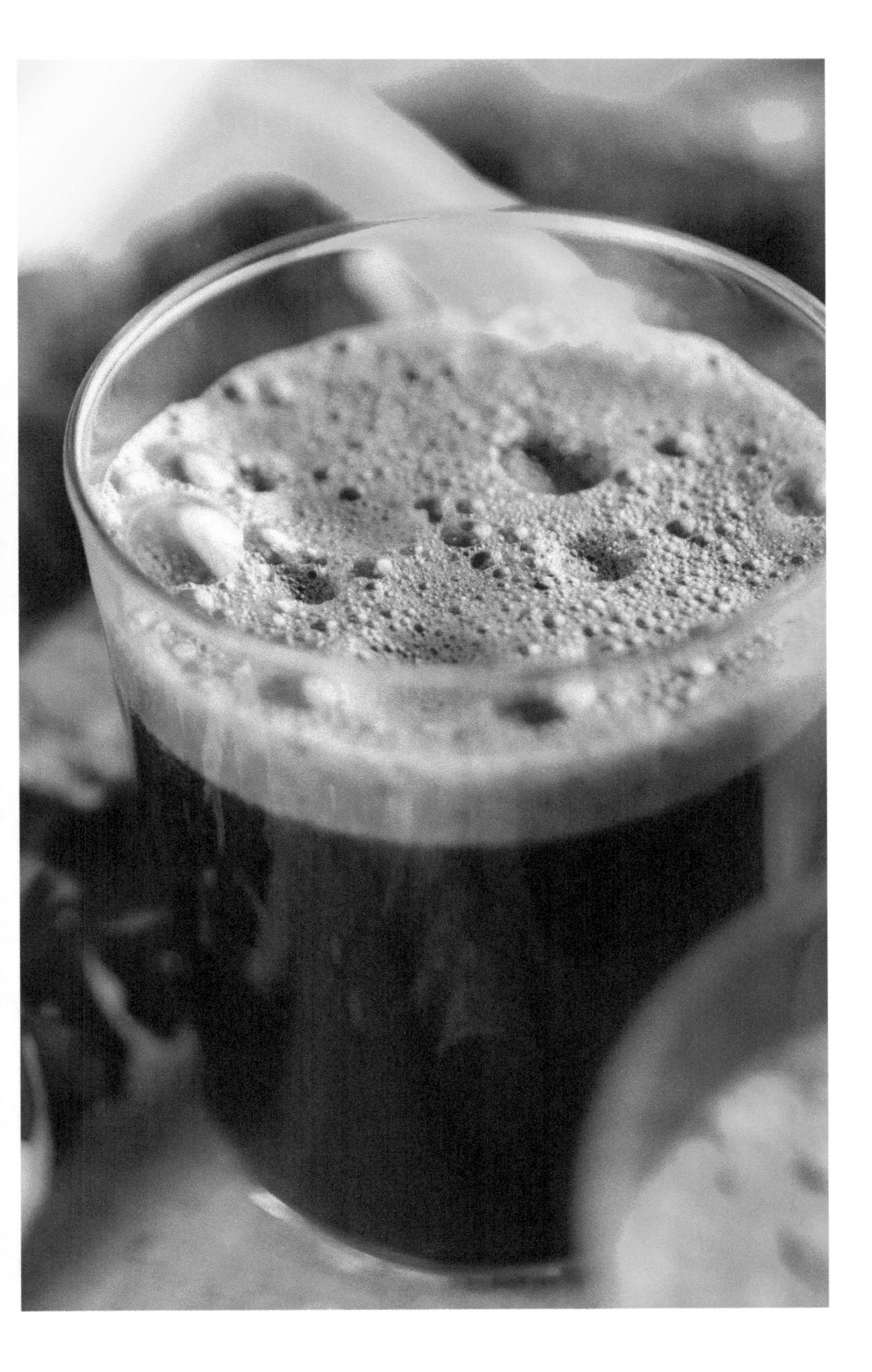

Jolly Green Giant Juice

SERVES 3

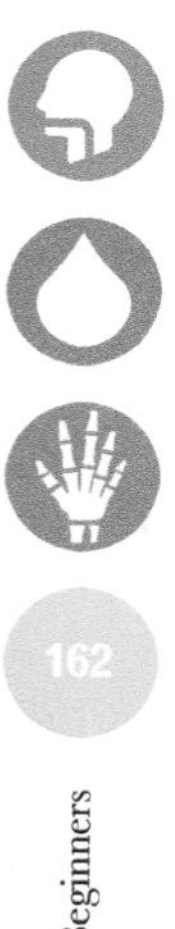

This juice with gigantic flavor and nutrients will leave you feeling lean and mean. Packed with vitamin-loaded ingredients like broccoli and romaine lettuce, this juice is more than just a beverage—it is fuel for your body.

4 LARGE STALKS CELERY
2 MEDIUM HEADS BROCCOLI
2 MEDIUM APPLES
½ HEAD ROMAINE LETTUCE
½ LEMON

1. Peel, cut, deseed, and/or chop the ingredients as needed.
2. Place a container under the juicer's spout.
3. Feed the ingredients one at a time, in the order listed, through the juicer.
4. Stir the juice and pour into glasses to serve.

Beets Me Blend

SERVES 3

If you have ever had beets, you may have been turned off by their dark purple color and strong odor. In this recipe, the beet flavor is disguised by the sweetness of apple juice and the fresh kick of ginger.

2 MEDIUM BEETS
1 LARGE HEAD BROCCOLI
1 BUNCH KALE LEAVES
½ BUNCH ASPARAGUS
1 MEDIUM APPLE
½-INCH PIECE GINGERROOT

1. Peel, cut, deseed, and/or chop the ingredients as needed.
2. Place a container under the juicer's spout.
3. Feed the ingredients one at a time, in the order listed, through the juicer.
4. Stir the juice and pour into glasses to serve.

Simply Sweet Green Juice

SERVES 3

Bok choy is a common ingredient in Asian cuisine, but in this recipe it provides both flavor and a variety of phytonutrients. Bok choy is an excellent source of fiber and antioxidants, which combine to provide anti-cancer and cholesterol-reducing benefits.

1 HEAD BABY BOK CHOY
1 SMALL HEAD BROCCOLI
1 MEDIUM CUCUMBER
½ MEDIUM ZUCCHINI
1 KIWI
1 MEDIUM APPLE
1 CLOVE GARLIC

1. Peel, cut, deseed, and/or chop the ingredients as needed.
2. Place a container under the juicer's spout.
3. Feed the ingredients one at a time, in the order listed, through the juicer.
4. Stir the juice and pour into glasses to serve.

Lean, Mean Green Juice

SERVES 2

Leafy greens like kale and Swiss chard are packed with vitamin K, calcium, and iron. They are also some of the most nutrient-dense vegetables in existence, which means you get all the benefits for very few calories!

4 LARGE CURLY KALE LEAVES
4 LARGE SWISS CHARD LEAVES
2 LARGE CARROTS
½ SMALL HEAD BROCCOLI
1 MEDIUM APPLE

1. Peel, cut, deseed, and/or chop the ingredients as needed.
2. Place a container under the juicer's spout.
3. Feed the ingredients one at a time, in the order listed, through the juicer.
4. Stir the juice and pour into glasses to serve.

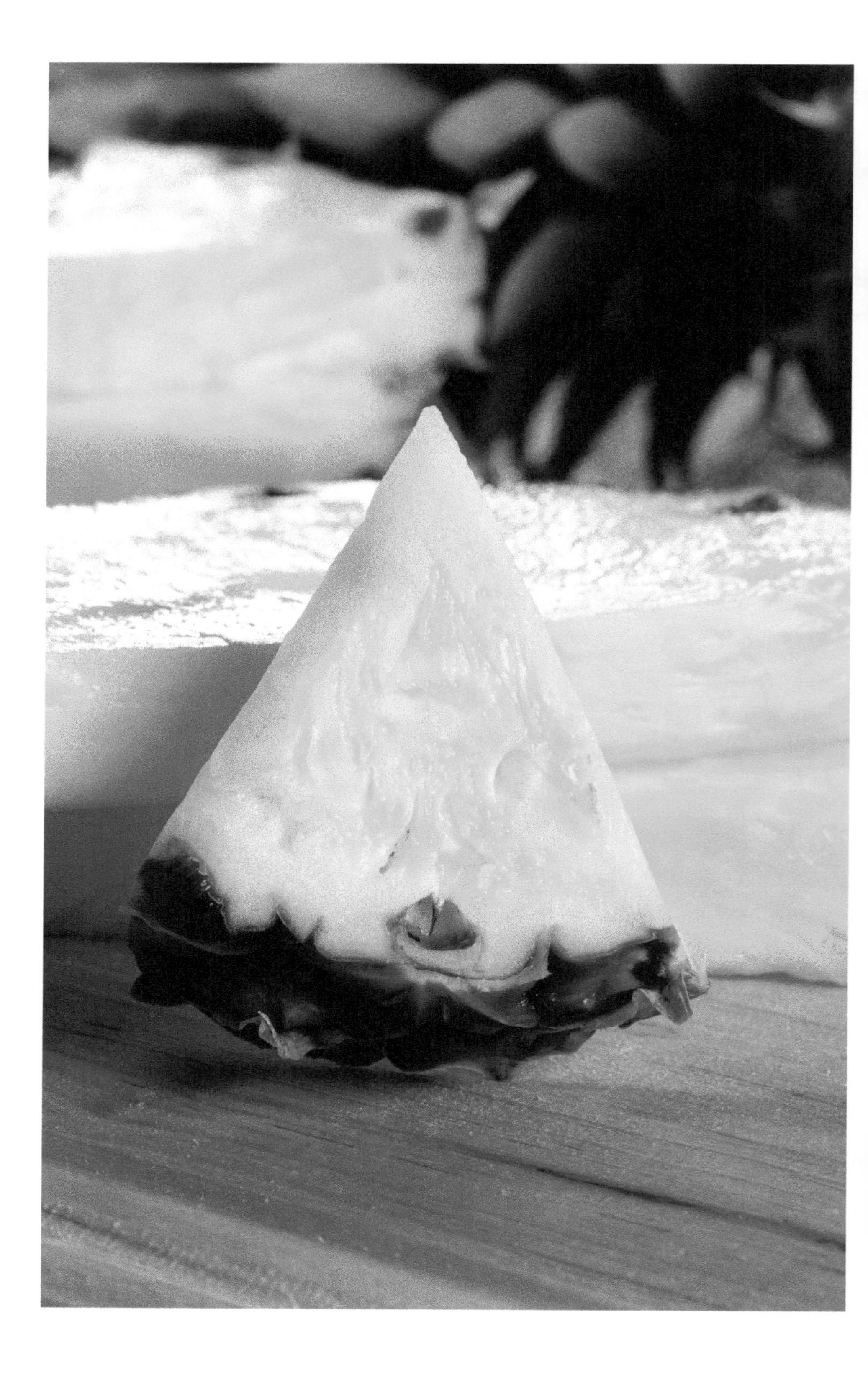

Green Goddess Juice

SERVES 2

Feel like a goddess (or god!) after drinking this delightful green juice. Full of healthy vitamins and minerals, it will leave you feeling utterly refreshed.

4 LARGE KALE LEAVES
1 CUP PINEAPPLE
½ BUNCH SPINACH LEAVES
1 MEDIUM APPLE

1. Peel, cut, deseed, and/or chop the ingredients as needed.
2. Place a container under the juicer's spout.
3. Feed the ingredients one at a time, in the order listed, through the juicer.
4. Stir the juice and pour into glasses to serve.

Get-Up-and-Go Juice

SERVES 2

This vitamin-packed energy juice is full of the nutrients you need to start your day off right. Lightly sweetened with apple juice and kiwis, this beverage is everything you could ever ask for in the morning.

4 LARGE COLLARD GREEN LEAVES
2 MEDIUM APPLES
2 RIPE KIWIS
1 SMALL HEAD BROCCOLI
1 CLOVE GARLIC

1. Peel, cut, deseed, and/or chop the ingredients as needed.
2. Place a container under the juicer's spout.
3. Feed the ingredients one at a time, in the order listed, through the juicer.
4. Stir the juice and pour into glasses to serve.

Sweet and Simple Green Juice

SERVES 2

You may be surprised to see dandelion greens as an ingredient in this recipe. Dandelion greens are actually a great source of vitamin K, which is essential for blood and bone health. These greens also support healthy liver and gallbladder function.

½ BUNCH SPINACH LEAVES
½ BUNCH DANDELION GREENS
2 LARGE CARROTS
1 SMALL APPLE
1 SMALL PEAR

1. Peel, cut, deseed, and/or chop the ingredients as needed.
2. Place a container under the juicer's spout.
3. Feed the ingredients one at a time, in the order listed, through the juicer.
4. Stir the juice and pour into glasses to serve.

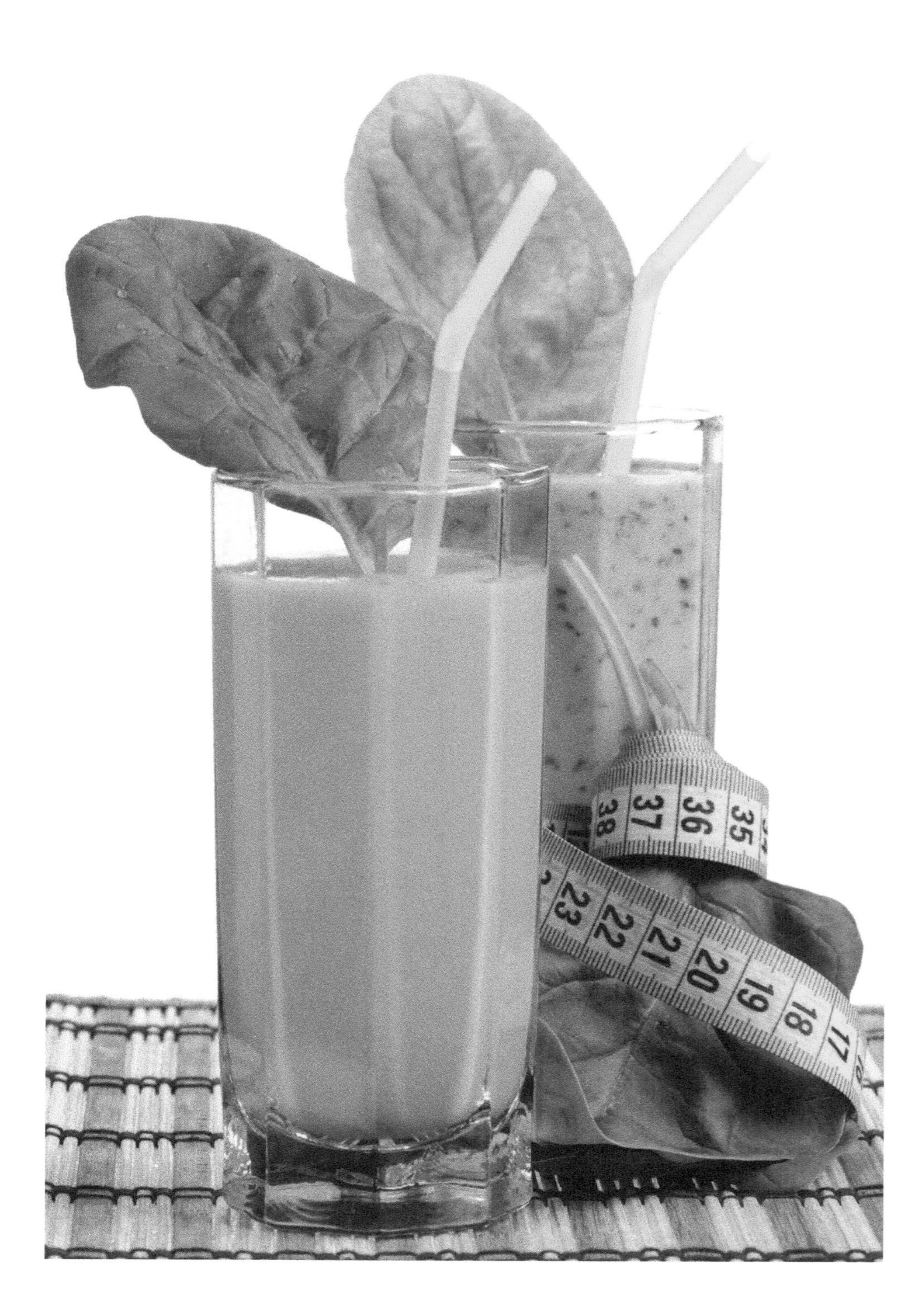

Conclusion

"Full of raw, seasonal produce, green juice is rich in vitamins, minerals, enzymes, and amino acids to nourish our insides for healthy skin, hair, nails, and teeth. And because it's in an easy-to-drink juice form, it's both quickly digested and absorbed with minimal effort by our bodies—meaning you get more bang for your buck, without having to eat eight cups of salad for breakfast!"

—NICOLE TEH, THE BEAUTY BEAN

Whether you are looking to lose weight, detoxify your body, or simply improve your health, juicing is the way to go. You are undoubtedly familiar with the saying "an apple a day keeps the doctor away" and other clichés encouraging the consumption of fresh fruits and vegetables. We are only human, though, and sometimes we get bored with eating the same foods, especially the very healthy ones. If it has become a challenge to fit your daily servings of fruit and vegetables into your routine, juicing is the perfect solution. You can get an entire salad's worth of fresh produce into a single glass of sip-able juice.

Not only is juicing quick and easy, but it is also good for you! By replacing unhealthy meals with fresh-pressed juices that are loaded with vitamins and minerals, you can significantly improve your overall health. Once you stop loading down your body with toxins and additives, your body will begin to efficiently process nutrients, resulting in healthier hair, skin, nails, and organs. Additionally, you are also likely to experience improved digestion, and if it is your goal, healthy and sustainable weight loss. Juicing is a wonderful option for the whole family, so try out some of the delicious recipes in this book together and improve your health today.

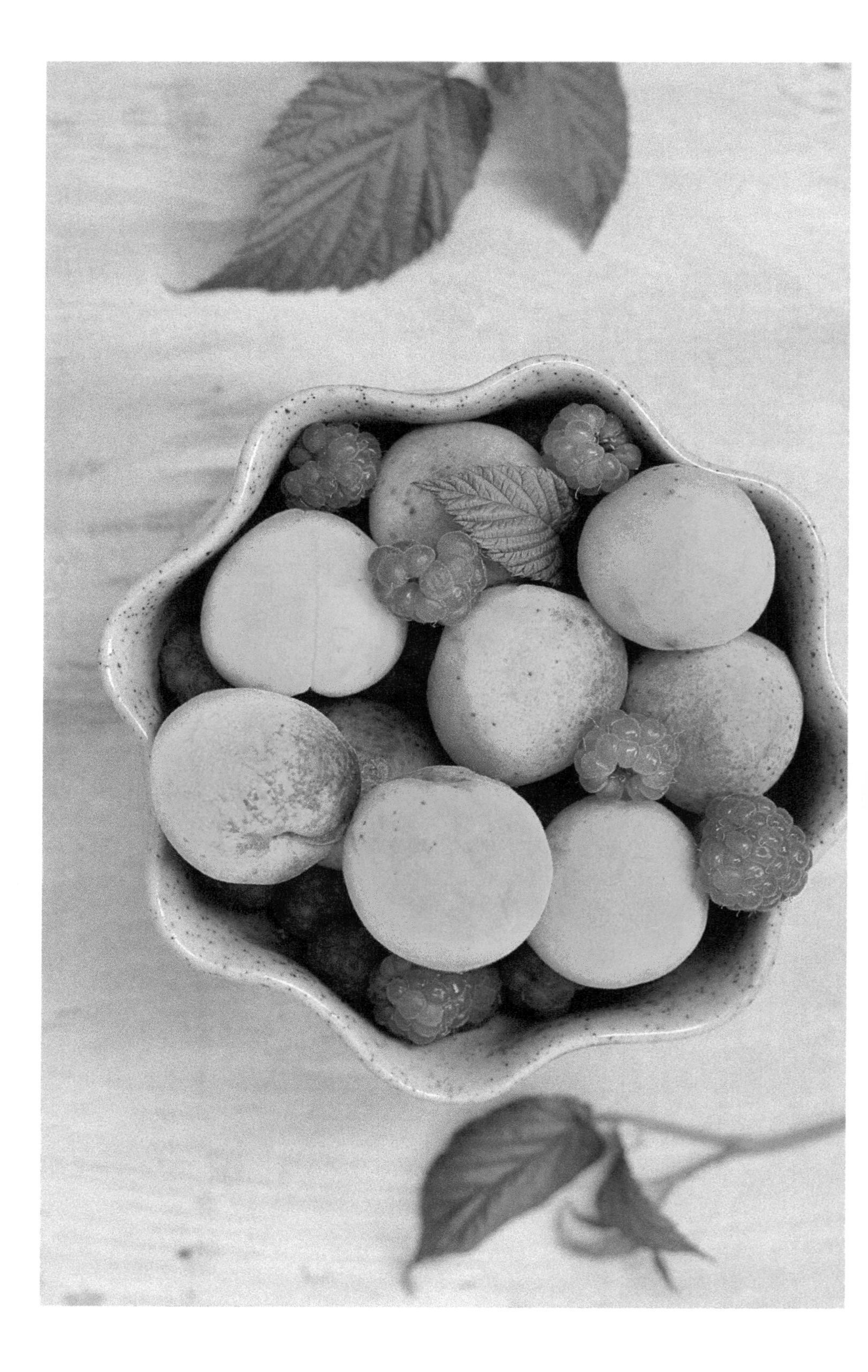

Glossary

Anthocyanins: a type of antioxidant pigment found in blood oranges, berries, radishes, and other produce.

Antioxidants: molecules that prevent other molecules from oxidizing. Antioxidants protect cells from damage by free radicals and may also help prevent cancer and other chronic diseases.

Basal metabolic rate (BMR): the minimum number of calories your body requires on a daily basis to maintain necessary functions.

BPA (bisphenol A): a synthetic chemical compound found in plastic that can cause serious health problems.

Centrifugal juicer: utilizes a grated basket that acts as a spinning blade, grinding the produce and extracting the juice.

Chlorella: a type of alga that is rich in a variety of nutrients, including protein, chlorophyll, iron, zinc, and vitamin B12.

Choline: a B-complex vitamin found in spinach that supports healthy cognitive function.

Detoxification: the flushing out or removal of harmful substances, like toxins, from the body.

Evolutionary discordance: occurs when a previously stable environment to which a species has adapted drastically and permanently changes without subsequent genetic changes in the species.

Fasting: the act of abstaining from food, liquid, or both for a defined period of time.

Flavonoid: a type of powerful antioxidant that can help repair damage caused by free radicals.

Juice cleanse: also known as a juice fast, a cleanse involves consuming nothing but fruit and vegetable juices for a predetermined length of time.

Juicer: a kitchen appliance that extracts the juice from fresh fruits and vegetables by various means. There are three types of juicers: centrifugal, masticating, and triturating.

Masticating juicer: a motor-driven appliance that works by kneading and grinding the produce in the feed chute, squeezing the juice out into a container.

Pectin: a soluble fiber that may help flush toxic heavy metals from the body.

Phytochemicals: also called phytonutrients, are compounds that naturally occur in plants and have biological significance (i.e. antioxidants).

Probiotics: living microorganisms that help to restore and improve healthy digestive function.

Quercetin: an antioxidant that helps to reduce LDL (bad) cholesterol levels.

Spirulina: a type of alga that is rich in both protein and essential amino acids.

Triturating juicer: also called a twin-gear juicer, it utilizes a two-step juicing process: when produce is fed through, it is first crushed and then it is pressed.

Whey powder: a nutritional supplement made from the proteins isolated from milk.

References

Carrera-Bastos et al, "The Western Diet and Lifestyle and Diseases of Civilization." *Research Reports in Clinical Cardiology*, 2011.

Cordain et al, "Origins and Evolution of the Western Diet: Health Implications for the 21st Century." *The American Society for Clinical Nutrition*, 2005. **http://ajcn.nutrition.org/content/81/2/341.full**

"Fruit Nutrition Facts." Nutrition-and-You.com. **www.nutrition-and-you.com/fruit-nutrition.html**

"Lifestyle Diseases." *Natural Health Perspective*. **http://naturalhealthperspective.com/home/civilization.html**

Vale, Jason. "A–Z of Ailments." Juice Master USA. **www.juicemaster.com/us/juice-therapy/a-to-z-ailments**

"Vegetable Nutrition Facts." Nutrition-and-You.com. **www.nutrition-and-you.com/vegetable-nutrition.html**

Nutritional Information Charts

NUTRITIONAL INFORMATION FOR FRUITS

SERVING SIZE = 100G

Food Name	Calories	Protein (grams)	Carbs (grams)	Fat (grams)	Fiber (grams)
Apple	50	0.26	13.81	0.17	2.4
Avocado	160	2.00	8.53	14.60	6.7
Banana	90	1.09	22.84	0.33	2.6
Blackberry	43	1.39	9.61	0.49	5.3
Black Cherry	50	1.00	12.18	0.30	1.6
Blood Orange	50	0.00	11.00	0.00	2.0
Blueberry	57	0.74	14.49	0.33	2.4
Cantaloupe	34	0.84	8.60	0.19	0.9
Grape	69	0.72	18.00	0.16	0.9
Grapefruit	42	0.77	10.70	0.14	1.7
Kiwi	61	1.00	14.66	0.52	3.0
Lemon	29	1.10	9.32	0.30	2.8
Lime	30	1.00	11.00	0.00	3.0
Mango	70	0.50	17.00	0.27	1.8
Melon	30	0.60	7.60	0.15	0.4
Orange	47	0.94	11.75	0.12	2.4
Papaya	39	0.61	9.81	0.14	1.8
Passion Fruit	97	2.20	23.40	0.70	10.4
Peach	39	0.91	9.54	0.25	1.5
Pear	58	0.38	13.81	0.12	3.1
Pineapple	50	0.54	13.52	0.12	1.4
Pomegranate	83	1.67	18.70	1.17	4.0
Raspberry	52	1.20	11.94	0.65	6.5
Strawberry	32	0.67	7.70	0.30	2.0
Tangerine	53	0.81	13.34	0.31	1.8

NUTRITIONAL INFORMATION FOR VEGETABLES

SERVING SIZE = 100G

Food Name	Calories	Protein (grams)	Carbs (grams)	Fat (grams)	Fiber (grams)
Arugula	25	2.58	3.65	0.66	1.6
Asparagus	20	2.20	3.38	0.12	2.1
Beet	45	1.61	9.56	0.17	2.8
Bell Pepper	31	0.99	6.03	0.30	2.1
Bok Choy	13	1.50	2.18	0.20	1.0 mg
Broccoli	34	2.82	6.64	0.37	2.6
Brussels Sprout	43	3.38	8.95	0.30	3.8
Cabbage	25	1.30	5.80	0.10	2.5 mg
Carrot	41	0.93	9.58	0.24	2.8
Cauliflower	25	1.92	4.97	0.28	2.0
Celery	16	1.00	3.00	0.00	2.0
Cilantro	23	2.00	4.00	1.00	3.0
Collard Greens	30	2.45	5.69	0.42	3.6
Cucumber	15	0.65	3.63	0.11	0.5
Dandelion Greens	45	3.00	9.00	1.00	4.0
Fennel	32	1.24	7.29	0.20	3.1
Garlic	149	6.00	33.00	0.00	2.0
Ginger	80	2.00	18.00	1.00	2.0
Kale	50	3.30	10.01	0.70	2.0
Mint	44	3.00	8.00	1.00	7.0
Parsley	36	3.00	6.00	1.00	3.0
Parsnip	75	1.20	18.00	0.30	4.9
Pumpkin	26	1.00	6.50	0.1	0.5
Romaine Lettuce	15	1.36	2.79	0.15	1.3
Spinach	23	2.86	3.63	0.39	2.2
Summer Squash	16	1.00	3.00	0.00	1.0
Sweet Potato	86	1.60	20.1	0.05	3.0
Swiss Chard	19	3.27	3.74	0.20	1.6
Tomato	18	0.90	3.90	0.20	1.2
Zucchini	17	1.21	3.11	0.32	1.0

NUTRITIONAL INFORMATION FOR ADDITIVES

SERVING SIZE = 1oz/28g

Food Name	Calories	Protein (grams)	Carbs (grams)	Fat (grams)	Fiber (grams)
Aloe Vera (juice)	2	0.00	1.00	0.00	0.0
Chlorella	81	16.00	7.00	2.00	1.0
Flaxseed	150	5.00	8.00	12.00	8.0
Flaxseed Oil	248	0.00	0.00	28.00	0.0
Hempseed	162	10.0	2.00	13.00	1.0
Herbal Extracts	N / A	N / A	N / A	N / A	N / A
Probiotic Capsules	N / A	N / A	N / A	N / A	N / A
Spirulina (dried)	81	16.00	7.00	2.00	1.0
Vitamin B12	N / A	N / A	N / A	N / A	N / A
Wheatgrass	7	0.00	1.00	0.00	0.0
Whey Powder	96	3.00	21.00	0.00	0.0

Conversion Tables

OVEN TEMPERATURES	
CELSIUS (C)	FAHRENHEIT (F)
120	250
150	300
180	355
200	400
220	450

VOLUME EQUIVALENTS	
METRIC	IMPERIAL (APPROXIMATE)
20 ML	½ FL OZ
60 ML	2 FL OZ
80 ML	3 FL OZ
125 ML	4½ FL OZ
160 ML	5½ FL OZ
180 ML	6 FL OZ
250 ML	9 FL OZ
375 ML	13 FL OZ
500 ML	18 FL OZ
750 ML	1½ PINTS
1 LITRE	1¾ PINTS

WEIGHT EQUIVALENTS	
METRIC	IMPERIAL (APPROXIMATE)
10 G	⅓ OZ
50 G	2 OZ
80 G	3 OZ
100 G	3½ OZ
150 G	5 OZ
175 G	6 OZ
250 G	9 OZ
375 G	13 OZ
500 G	1 LB
750 G	1⅔ LB
1 KG	2 LB

CUP AND SPOON CONVERSIONS	
5 ML	1 TEASPOON
20 ML	1 TABLESPOON
60 ML	¼ CUP
80 ML	⅓ CUP
125 ML	½ CUP
160 ML	⅔ CUP
180 ML	¾ CUP
250 ML	1 CUP

Index

C

D

E

F

G

H

I

J

Q

R

S

T

U

V

W

Y

Z

CPSIA information can be obtained
at www.ICGtesting.com
Printed in the USA
BVHW091330200221
600431BV00010B/14